MW01716905

Super Bowl Fit

Mainstreaming Chinese Medicine & Acupuncture

Homa Sajadian Sikon L.Ac., Dipl. O.M.

Table of Contents

Introduction

You may wonder what Traditional Chinese Medicine and acupuncture have to do with the Super Bowl... Besides the fact that many Super Bowl players are avid acupuncture fans, including Tom Brady, the winner of seven Super Bowls.

As a Traditional Chinese Medicine practitioner since 2008, I am enchanted by the healing powers of acupuncture every day. Acupuncture harnesses and refocuses the body's own healing powers to treat physical and emotional ailments, and it does so safely and without any side effects. Acupuncture restores balance and makes you feel centered. Acupuncture calms the nerves and helps you shed that extra, uneasy static that you feel but can't quite describe. Acupuncture helps you feel an overall state of well-being that is hard to describe unless you experience it firsthand. Acupuncture is so remarkably effective in restoring health and vitality that it makes me wonder why more people don't know about it and embrace it.

And here's how this powerful medicine ties into the Super Bowl: If mainstream television commercials truly reflected the benefits of a product or service, there would be half-time Super Bowl commercials about Traditional Chinese Medicine and acupuncture, as nothing gets more mainstream in the U.S. than the Super Bowl. Who doesn't love a great Super Bowl party, the game, the excitement, the half-time shows, and all the commercials?

The advantages of Traditional Chinese Medicine and acupuncture are so incredible that they should be advertised during the Super Bowl for the benefit of all. Wouldn't you want to know how to truly feel your best? Wouldn't you want to feel better than OK and be Super Bowl fit?

Given that a typical Super Bowl ad cost upwards of 6 million U.S. dollars for 30 seconds in 2023, the likelihood of ever having a half-time commercial promoting acupuncture for your priceless health and vitality is very slim. Traditional Chinese Medicine doesn't make any corporations rich, and that is why it is not advertised in the mainstream media. Traditional Chinese Medicine is not only remarkably effective in restoring health and vitality; it is also a very low-cost system of medicine with potentially millions of dollars in cost savings.

The goal of this book is to demystify and introduce acupuncture to the mainstream, specifically for those who are proactive about their health and vitality. The book covers the benefits of acupuncture without relying too much on unfamiliar or abstract terms such as qi, yin, and yang.

Moreover, you will learn about acupuncture as a true form of healthcare, not merely sick care. Sick care is physically, emotionally, and financially draining, but sadly, it is currently the norm in society. Once you discover the amazing restorative powers of acupuncture, I hope you will come to see acupuncture as something like a family dental practice that serves people of all ages and conditions in the community. Regular acupuncture treatments and tune-ups as preventative maintenance are very similar to routine dental checkups and cleanings.

As promised, we won't dwell on a lot of complicated historical and philosophical discussions in this book. At the same time, we will meet Otzi the Iceman, the hunter-gatherer who froze in the Alps five thousand years ago with evidence of acupuncture marks on his back along the way. We will also see how analogies with modern technologies, such as Wi-Fi and cellular networks, can help us better understand some acupuncture concepts.

I can speak for myself and my colleagues when I say that, as acupuncture practitioners, we truly care about our craft and the profound positive impact it has on each of our patients' quality of life. Most of us, especially in the West, were not born into a lineage of acupuncturists, nor did we daydream of becoming an acupuncturist as children. Our journey started with our own health challenges, which led to life-changing personal experiences with Traditional Chinese Medicine. With renewed hope in our own well-being, years of studying and the acquired in-depth knowledge, we feel compelled to help others. I hope I have piqued your interest to join me in this easy-going yet profoundly eye-opening journey to discover a complementary system of medicine that can help millions of people around the world, including you and your loved ones, to be hopeful and in better control of your health and well-being at any age.

Chapter 1:

A Bit of History

Otzi, the prehistoric iceman, was surprisingly in great physical shape for his age when he was frozen in time by the fate of an arrow 5,300 years ago. Otzi had 61 tattoos around his body, all plain stripes with two crosses, some with striking correspondence to common acupuncture points used today. He was also a fan of herbology, as evidenced by the medicinal mushrooms he had eaten shortly before he froze to death. Otzi was perfectly preserved in ice when he was discovered in 1991 by hikers in the Alps.

We have come to think of acupuncture points as being inseparably associated with Traditional Chinese Medicine, but the use of acupuncture points may have been more widespread in ancient times than we know. Scientists think Otzi's tattoos were produced by making small incisions on the skin and then rubbing them with charcoal. The experts believe the markings are some kind of medicinal therapy because of their appearance and location on the body. They could have been made to treat the disease that Otzi was suffering from, including joint and spinal problems (Ghose, 2018).

Possible evidence of the use of acupuncture points in the past has been discovered in other parts of the world. Acupuncture points could have been a component of ancient Andean medical practices, as evidenced by the tattoos that an archaeologist team found on a woman who was 1,000 years old. They discovered 12 overlapping circles on the woman's neck that resembled patterns of therapeutic acupuncture points commonly used today to treat neck pain (Manohar, 2010).

There are still people in remote parts of the world who practice rudimentary forms of acupuncture, breaking the skin with sharp instruments to heal illness. They include South Africa's Bantu people and some people in far-off areas of Brazil and the circumpolar North. What makes Traditional Chinese Medicine unique is that every single acupuncture point, its actions, indications, and precise anatomical location were meticulously documented in texts dating back over 2,000 years. The textbooks I used to study Traditional Chinese Medicine are the modern versions of these ancient texts that have evolved and survived the test of time for thousands of years.

How I Discovered Acupuncture—a Personal Journey

I was in my 20s when my sister became a licensed acupuncturist. I saw her treat family and friends with chronic pain. As a healthy and active young person blissfully unfamiliar with pain, I was neither drawn to acupuncture nor even slightly curious about it at that time. I studied Electrical Engineering as an undergraduate and received my Master's of Science in Operations Research and Management Science. I had always been fascinated with space, so I went on to work on multibillion-dollar communications satellite systems.

Growing up in Washington, D.C., I had seasonal hay fever treated with over-the-counter allergy medications. The season was short, and suffering from allergies was just an inconvenient couple of months per year. Eventually, my job took me to San Diego and then Los Angeles in my early 30s, and that's when I started experiencing health issues.

My first personal experience with acupuncture came after a rowing injury. It was a dark and cold morning when I felt a painful pop in my lower back. I was lifting the boat when my crewmate behind me suddenly let go of the boat. Anyone who has experienced back pain can attest to how physically and emotionally draining it is, in addition to being painful. My doctor advised resting, icing, and pain medication, none of which seemed to help my situation. That is when I resorted to trying acupuncture. I received my very first acupuncture treatment on my couch in my living room while my sister, Sepideh Lackpour, an accomplished acupuncturist herself, was visiting for the afternoon. I recall being surprised by how uneventful the experience was. I didn't feel the needles and just laid on my couch, enjoying the afternoon sun through the window, for about half an hour.

The next morning, I felt a renewed sense of energy and vitality, though my back still continued to ache. The renewed energy was quite different from drinking a cup of coffee or having a good night's sleep. I just felt "optimized," clear-headed, and energetic in a balanced way.

While that first treatment didn't dramatically help my back, I was intrigued by the experience and my response to the treatment. I asked my sister if acupuncture could possibly be the reason why I felt such great energy the next morning. She responded, "Yes, I just noticed you were fatigued, so I thought I'd give you a boost." Like tuning a violin, acupuncture fine-tuned me. It shook off the static energy that I had been experiencing since feeling that pop in my lower back. It calmed my nerves and relaxed my muscles. I no longer felt drained physically and emotionally from the back pain. It harmonized my body and mind and eventually healed my back.

Several months after moving to Los Angeles, I started getting sick a lot. I would lose my voice regularly and catch every cold or flu that was going around in the office, and I wasn't able to just push through. I missed work at my new job and canceled social engagements often. I started seeing my doctor regularly for courses of antibiotics, inhalers, steroid nasal sprays, and whatnot. After months of treatment for recurrent upper respiratory infections, my doctor recommended that I see an allergist. I tested positive for everything in my new environment, from dust and mold to olive and eucalyptus trees and cat and dog dander. They put me on allergy medication, gave me a rescue inhaler and a maintenance inhaler, and recommended that I start allergy shots. I started noticing TV commercials for a few of my medications, followed by "ask your doctor about the XYZ medication," and then, a long list of side effects blurred out very fast, some of which seemed a lot worse than what I was experiencing and having allergies.

As an engineer, I was clueless about my body and how to maintain my health. I ate well, exercised, and relied on my doctor if anything felt off. As an engineer, I was also a problem solver and innately knew that taking medications for the rest of my life or moving elsewhere was not the solution. After all, I had moved to Los Angeles from San Diego, where I was surrounded by olive and eucalyptus trees, dander, and dust without any problems. My doctor's response was that people could develop allergies later in life. I asked if there were any options other than taking the pills, getting allergy shots, or moving, and I was told those were my only options.

Having had that aha moment experience with acupuncture months earlier, I turned to Traditional Chinese Medicine. I received regular acupuncture treatments and took the recommended herbal formulas while continuing with the medications. I felt empowered and hopeful about my health as I navigated between Traditional Chinese and Western medicines. I was able to successfully wean myself from the allergy medication and inhalers within several months. I learned that while I had always been sensitive to allergens in my environment, such as when I had occasional hay fever in Washington, DC, the less-than-desirable air quality in my new environment had weakened my defense system so much that I could no longer tolerate these allergens. With the help of Traditional Chinese Medicine's herbal formulas and acupuncture, my defense system regained its strength over time. With my newly acquired knowledge about my body and with lifestyle and diet modifications, I was able to keep strong so that I no longer needed to rely on allergy medication.

I was fascinated with the idea of treating not just the symptoms but the root cause of ailments, so much so that I decided to leave my successful career in aerospace engineering and follow my calling to study Traditional Chinese Medicine. In 2004, I left the world of satellite communications and went back to school for a 4-year master's program in Traditional Chinese Medicine, shifting my attention from orbits deep in outer space to meridians orbiting within the human body.

In 2008, I graduated Magna Cum Laude from Emperor's College, which was founded in 1983 and is one of the oldest acupuncture schools in the nation. I have been a licensed practitioner of Traditional Chinese Medicine ever since, treating patients from all walks of life and from around the world at luxury spas, gyms, community clinics, cruise ships, and in my local community.

Over the years, my problem-solving skills and engineering background have greatly assisted me in getting to the root cause of ailments and helping my patients achieve optimal health. I have witnessed first-hand how each of us is truly a microcosm of our environment, associating acupuncture meridians with space orbits. Instead of focusing just on symptoms, I view a person as a whole and treat the root cause of a disorder. I utilize acupuncture/acupressure, herbal Medicine, and coaching in nutrition, exercise, and lifestyle recommendations based on the fundamentals of Traditional Chinese Medicine. I strive to empower my patients to tune in and listen to their bodies to restore their health and vitality.

Health and vitality are the norms and the natural state we are meant to be in. While visiting Michelangelo's masterpiece, David, in Florence many years ago, I stood in awe of his process as described by the tour guide. Michelangelo didn't carve a figure out of the stone, but he revealed the statue that was hidden within it. Traditional Chinese Medicine helps reveal your health buried under the debris of daily stressors, viruses, poor diet, physical and emotional trauma, and the environment.

The Mythical Father of Chinese Medicine

In ancient China, acupuncture was regarded as an intervention of the utmost importance from ancient times. It was so revered that successive ruling dynasties required the presence of expert acupuncture clinicians in their courts and established educational institutions that were solely devoted to acupuncture.

The most important figure in Traditional Chinese Medicine's history is the legendary Yellow Emperor, also known as the Mythical Father of Chinese Medicine. The legend has it that he lived in the period of the Warring States (475–221 BC), but his biography is clouded by so much mystery that no historian can be certain when he lived or if he even existed at all.

According to legend, the Yellow Emperor's mother was impregnated by a whirling light that originated from the star constellation known as the Plough. He was born after a pregnancy that lasted twenty-four months and could engage in profound philosophical discourse only a few days after his birth, an unlikely character indeed.

The Yellow Emperor's *Classic of Internal Medicine*, or the *Inner Canon of the Yellow Emperor*, is the earliest and most important text focusing on acupuncture or Traditional Chinese Medicine, dating back to 2200 years ago. The book is written in the style of a conversation that takes place between the emperor and his physician. In this conversation, the emperor asks his doctor questions regarding the nature of health, illness, and therapy.

According to historians, the Yellow Emperor's *Classic of Internal Medicine* is a compilation of the works of multiple authors over time. Part mythical and perhaps part historical, the Yellow Emperor is significant because, even in the present period, Traditional Chinese Medicine practitioners continue to find the book useful as a reference work. It is probably the oldest living medical literature and has been quite influential in the evolution of Traditional Chinese Medicine for over two millennia.

A recurring thread throughout acupuncture's fascinating history has been its evolution. Every Grand Master of Chinese medicine added their findings to what had come before, which changed how people viewed acupuncture. Acupuncture has endured throughout history, surviving many cultures, beliefs, and shifts in how people view healthcare.

Acupuncture in the United States

The first introduction of acupuncture into the U.S. dates back to 1825, when Franklin Bache, a physician, and great-grandson of Benjamin Franklin, published an academic paper on its benefits. In the early 20th century, Dr. William Osler recommended acupuncture for treating low back pain in his highly reputable *Principles and Practice of Medicine*, but it was a July 1971 story by journalist James Reston in the *New York Times* that was largely responsible for the surge in popularity of acupuncture in the U.S.

While covering a visit by Secretary of State Henry Kissinger to China, Reston underwent an emergency appendectomy in a Beijing hospital and received acupuncture treatment afterward. His observations regarding acupuncture's success in relieving his post-operative pain sparked interest in the U.S., which has since grown.

A Rose by Any Other Name

Before diving any deeper, let's briefly touch upon a question that may cause some confusion among readers. In daily usage and scientific literature, Traditional Chinese Medicine has been variably referred to as Oriental Medicine, Traditional Chinese Medicine, Traditional Asian Medicine, or simply Chinese Medicine, among other names. We will stick with Traditional Chinese Medicine throughout this book. They all denote essentially the same system of medicine that includes a comprehensive and methodical diagnosis, identifying the root cause, and delivering treatment using acupuncture, herbal formulas, nutrition, and other means, which we will cover later in the book. A practitioner of this comprehensive system of medicine is typically referred to as an acupuncturist, even though acupuncture is only one aspect of the medicine they practice. For the sake of simplicity, the medicine itself is sometimes referred to as acupuncture. Nevertheless, as Shakespeare put it, "A rose by any other name would smell as sweet."

Chapter 2:

Unraveling the Mystery of Acupuncture

To many people, Traditional Chinese Medicine, in general, and acupuncture, in particular, appear as mysterious and perplexing subjects. There are so many myths and misconceptions going around that the simple truth is obscured: acupuncture is a recognized, reliable, accessible, and effective therapy that helps treat a wide range of common health and lifestyle problems. It restores balance and creates a wonderful sense of well-being. Misconceptions about acupuncture not only hold people back from enjoying its amazing benefits; they prevent some from ever considering it to begin with.

So let us debunk some common acupuncture myths and misconceptions. Here are 10 of the most widespread myths about acupuncture:

Myth #1: "Acupuncture is painful."

Top of the list, let's address the elephant in the room: the acupuncture needle. Contrary to popular belief, acupuncture needles are not painful. Often, people don't feel them at all. Most people's aversion to acupuncture is because of their experience with hypodermic needles. Acupuncture needles are very different from hypodermic needles used for injections. Acupuncture needles are incredibly small, some looking like cats' whiskers. You can fit many acupuncture needles inside a hypodermic needle. Hypodermic needles are sharp and hollow and are designed to cut through the body tissue and deliver or draw fluids. By contrast, acupuncture needles are solid and pliable; they are designed to glide. In the U.S., an acupuncture needle is a medical device regulated by the FDA. It is made of surgical stainless steel, is single-use, and is disposed of in a special medical sharps container after use.

Myth #2: "Acupuncture may cause scarring or marks."

No, acupuncture does not cause scarring when it is done by trained Traditional Chinese Medicine practitioners licensed to perform acupuncture. The acupuncture needle is very fine. It is not hollow and is not designed to cut like hypodermic needles. It is typically a superfine laser-cut surgical stainless steel needle with a rounded tip designed to glide between the cells so it does not injure the tissue or damage the skin. In fact, acupuncture is very helpful in treating both new and old scar tissue from a past injury or surgery.

Myth #3: "Acupuncture is just for treating pain."

Absolutely not! Acupuncture is a powerful treatment under the umbrella of Traditional Chinese Medicine. Today, acupuncture is recognized as a valid form of complementary medicine for treating a wide range of non-pain-related complaints, from autoimmune conditions and anxiety to vertigo and weight loss. Depending on your condition, acupuncture is used as a standalone treatment or as a complementary treatment in conjunction with conventional medical therapies. You don't even have to be sick or have a condition to receive acupuncture. Acupuncture is a preventative medicine as well, just like dentistry, which can be preventative in addition to treating dental problems. For example, a lot of times, athletes come in for an acupuncture session as a preventive measure to improve performance, prevent injury, and help with faster recovery from their training. People also come for their acupuncture to help with their immune systems or just to get a general tune-up for their general health. You may even get acupuncture to reduce the effects of jetlag and help harmonize your circadian rhythm, as was the case for this patient: "A nice experience straight after a very long plane flight from Australia. I feel relaxed and well-balanced. Thank you!"

Myth #4: "You should try acupuncture only as a last resort when all else fails."

Please don't wait that long. Acupuncture promotes circulation, reduces inflammation, and mobilizes your own stem cells to repair and heal your body. Healing is a process; the sooner you start treatment, the faster you will see results. The more chronic a condition, the longer the healing process, and as mentioned earlier, you don't even need to have a condition to get acupuncture. Prevention is the best form of medicine.

Myth #5: "You need a doctor's referral or a prescription for acupuncture."

Possibly, it depends on the state or country you live in. In California, Traditional Chinese Medicine practitioners are primary healthcare providers, so patients do not need a prescription unless required by their insurance company.

Myth #6: "Acupuncture can conflict with standard treatments such as cancer care or physical therapy."

Acupuncture does not interfere with any treatment. On the contrary, it often helps accelerate your benefits from whatever healing treatment modality you are using because it stimulates your body to repair and regenerate.

Myth #7: "I've heard people may get worse after an acupuncture treatment."

Occasionally, a patient may have increased symptoms after an acupuncture session, which people misinterpret as acupuncture worsening their condition. This situation is only temporary and is called the "healing crisis." A healing crisis may be a sign of detoxification in the body, or it may occur because your body is already fighting something—a virus, for example. Your energy level may drop after treatment because the body is using all its resources to fight off the virus or whatever it is fighting. It is best to continue the treatment course and support your body by not interrupting the healing process.

Myth #8: "Acupuncture is not good for autoimmune conditions because it boosts the immune system."

Acupuncture helps restore balance in the body and helps your immune system harmonize itself. This means that for those with a weakened immune system, treatments strengthen the body, and for those with autoimmunity, acupuncture attempts to restore balance in the immune system. There is considerable scientific evidence that acupuncture is beneficial for managing autoimmune diseases such as rheumatoid arthritis and inflammatory bowel disease (IBD).

Myth #9: "I tried acupuncture once, and it didn't work."

You may have stopped the treatment too early. It is like taking vitamin C— you don't just take it once and expect results from one dose of vitamin C. Acupuncture facilitates the healing process. Still, sufficient treatment is needed for it to take effect. In general, acute conditions can be fully treated in 1 to 3 sessions. More chronic conditions require more treatments, and you will taper down the frequency and number of treatments over time.

Myth #10: "You have to believe in acupuncture in order for it to work for you."

No, acupuncture works regardless of one's belief system, as clearly shown in veterinary acupuncture. It is widely used with pets, farm animals, and even animals in zoos across the world because it is so effective. Acupuncture has a real physiological impact on the body; it improves circulation, regulates hormones, calms the nerves, reduces inflammation, and facilitates healing, all regardless of one's belief system. An acupuncture skeptic wrote: "My first time with acupuncture. I was a complete agnostic. However, a series of treatments did, in fact, result in the elimination of chronic neck pain, and each session was more rewarding than the one before. The feeling of relaxation and well-being that follows each session is remarkable."

Chapter 3:

From Sick Care to Health Care

Acupuncture can be an excellent treatment for various illnesses, but it may be even better at preventing them. There is nothing new in this statement; Traditional Chinese Medicine has utilized acupuncture primarily as a powerful preventive tool for thousands of years. The reasons acupuncture was billed as a relief measure in the West are myriad and complex. Undoubtedly, this is, to a large extent, due to our propensity to prioritize disease treatment over prevention. It may also have something to do with the way acupuncture was introduced to the U.S. in the 20th century as a complementary therapy for post-surgery pain relief.

Whatever the reasons, perhaps now, more than ever, is the moment to expand our awareness from only curing disease to also promoting wellness, as preventing disease is much more efficient and cost-effective than waiting for it to strike. Traditional Chinese Medicine advises taking this course of action to maintain your health at its peak today and prevent disease patterns from developing in the future.

Sick Care Versus Health Care

As Americans, we can count ourselves fortunate to have access to the best healthcare system in the world, one that uses continually improving technologies to help us with a range of health issues. There are numerous publicly sponsored and privately financed insurance programs to pay for the cost of the patient's care in this system. These insurance plans cover and pay for the great majority of doctor visits, laboratory work, radiology and special test investigations, medication, and sometimes even limited complementary treatments such as acupuncture. However, rarely do these insurance plans cover preventive care or treatments that improve the patient's quality of life in the maintenance phase.

The most complex medical issues can be successfully treated in the U.S. However, the system as a whole was harshly criticized in a 2012 paper published in *The New England Journal of Medicine* for its insufficient focus on preventive measures. According to the authors, the healthcare system in the U.S. is a fragmented, task-based system that reimburses for "sick visits" intended to address acute conditions or acute exacerbations of chronic diseases. Economic incentives drive the overuse of such services by promoting procedural over cognitive tasks (such as surgery over behavior-change counseling) and specialists over primary care. In practice, these misaligned economic incentives disfavor successful prevention through health maintenance (Fani Marvasti & Stafford, 2012).

A decade later, a bias toward clinical action still governs how healthcare is delivered, even though the Affordable Care Act (ACA) aims to promote a more all-encompassing healthcare experience. The ACA requires nearly all health insurance plans to include specific categories of regular and preventative care. This is a solid base, especially for consumers who are in good health, but beyond these basic features, the main emphasis remains on treating diseases rather than preserving the health and well-being of the individual.

The current model of sick care revolves around doctors, lab tests, and prescription medications. Many doctors look forward to helping and treating patients with health issues when they graduate from medical school and start their practices, whether it is an illness, a medical emergency, or another serious health condition. However, crucial factors affecting a person's health do not receive sufficient attention in the sick care model. These factors include chronic repetitive strains as well as underlying social, emotional, and mental crises, which significantly impact health outcomes. In fact, these elements are mostly to blame for a person's physical diseases and health issues. Physical, physiological, nutritional, emotional, mental, and social stressors frequently accumulate in the body over time and cause the diseases that the "sick care" system then treats.

The current system is best suited to helping individuals who are in pain or ill. It is intended to help patients who have already reached a stage in which their body's defense mechanisms are no longer able to withstand the stresses being applied to them, and as a result, the symptoms of their condition, such as severe back pain from a herniated disc, high blood pressure, or thyroid problems, emerge and start to negatively impact their quality of life.

The World Health Organization (WHO) states that "health is a state of complete physical, mental, and social well-being and not merely the absence of disease or infirmity" (WHO, 1946). In this important statement, health is defined as more than merely the absence of illness or disease. Human beings are in a permanent state of flux between two opposite ends of a spectrum that characterizes health. Optimal health is at one end of the spectrum, and sickness and disease are at the other.

The current state of affairs profoundly distorts consumers' views of what is important in healthcare and what is not. Many Americans mistakenly believe that if a medical service is not covered by insurance schemes, it is not important or necessary. Therefore, people only spend a small amount of out-of-pocket money on preventative healthcare requirements. In effect, they rely mainly on the "sick care" model for their health. Imagine taking your car in only when the engine light goes on or if the routine service for your car is limited to inspecting the car and running diagnostics. A routine tune-up for your car is more than just a check-up; in contrast, the annual health physical for your most valuable and irreplaceable asset is typically limited to a check-up.

A paradigm shift in how we view health is crucial to moving away from our present sick care model and toward one that also incorporates a preventative health care strategy. People will almost certainly be heading toward sickness and moving further away from optimal health if they wait for major symptoms of illness and disease as the primary indicator of their overall state of health. Particularly in today's hectic society, one must actively pursue an optimal level of health if they don't want to move closer to the extreme end of the health spectrum because of their chronic lifestyle habits.

The Avoidable Burden of Sick Care

More than 75% of the money we spend on healthcare in the U.S. goes toward the management of potentially preventable chronic diseases. These illnesses, which are the main causes of death and disability in the country, leave behind fatalities that could have been avoided, lifelong disabilities, reduced quality of life, and huge healthcare expenses. The evidence is startling. Chronic diseases cause 7 out of 10 deaths in Americans each year. Nearly one in two people suffers from at least one chronic condition. About one-fourth of people with chronic illnesses have restrictions on daily activities. Chronic diseases and mental health are intimately associated. Chronic illnesses might worsen the symptoms of depression and vice versa (National Center for Chronic Disease Prevention and Health Promotion, 2009).

The public is aware of the size and severity of the chronic disease problem. In a survey, more than two-thirds of respondents felt that the American healthcare system should prioritize chronic illness prevention. More than four out of five people support public funding for such preventative initiatives.

The Human Cost of Sickness

Let's examine the primary diseases and health conditions that affect our country, such as heart disease, stroke, diabetes, and arthritis more closely (National Center for Chronic Disease Prevention and Health Promotion, 2009).

Heart Disease and Stroke: These diseases are among the leading causes of disability and continue to be the first and third leading causes of death, accounting for more than 30% of all deaths. One million Americans have stroke-related disabilities; many of them cannot walk or shower without assistance.

Diabetes: Nearly 24 million Americans have diabetes, and prediabetes puts an estimated 57 million more at an elevated risk of getting the disease. Diabetes is increasing in prevalence every day. According to current statistics, 1 in 3 Americans born in 2000 will get diabetes at some point in their lives. For individuals aged between 20 and 74, diabetes continues to be the main cause of kidney failure, non-traumatic lower-extremity amputations, and blindness.

Arthritis: Having arthritis creates unique obstacles to exercising and engaging in regular activity. This situation also obstructs efforts to treat and manage other chronic illnesses the individual may have. Racial and ethnic minorities are disproportionately affected by the incapacitating effects of arthritis. For instance, more African Americans than Whites reported having severe pain, as well as having activity and employment restrictions related to arthritis.

The Financial Cost of Preventable Diseases

Individuals, their families, and the country as a whole face enormous financial costs, not to mention the emotional and mental price, as a result of preventable chronic diseases. For instance, it was estimated that diabetes had direct medical expenditures of $116.0 billion in 2007. In 2009, cardiovascular disease and stroke claimed $313.8 billion in direct costs. The costs of these and other potentially preventable diseases continue to grow (National Center for Chronic Disease Prevention and Health Promotion, 2009).

The predicted increase in demand for family and professional caregivers, who are now present in one out of every five households, intensifies this trend. The expenses to families, companies, and communities are enormous, and the toll on caregivers' health and well-being is severe.

Stay Healthy Instead of Waiting for Illness to Strike

As a child, you may have read Dr. Seuss' book, *Oh, the Places You'll Go!*, where he says, "You have brains in your head. You have feet in your shoes. You can steer yourself in any direction you choose. You're on your own. And you know what you know. And YOU are the guy who'll decide where to go."

You can design your own life, and your decisions and actions now will eventually determine how your future will be shaped. Optimizing your health now can lay a strong foundation for your enjoyment and contentment as you move through life.

Health is not something that just happens. Although it may be true that some people are more predisposed to certain illnesses than others, maintaining good health requires effort. It requires wise choices, perseverance, and commitment. When you take charge of your health, it improves. But how should we go about it? We are all comfortable with our reactive health strategy, which involves waiting until a health problem arises before seeking medical assistance. However, it doesn't work in our best interest. If you are tired of waiting for excellent health and want to create it instead, you should start being proactive about it right now.

Why wait for symptoms to appear before treating them when you can try to avoid them? Preventive health entails caring for your body before problems arise. Prioritizing your health will help you build up your immunity and fend off illnesses. Making your health a priority can lengthen your life, improve your quality of life, and contribute to your overall well-being.

Unfortunately, most busy people rarely give proactive healthcare planning much thought. They only concentrate on seeking medical care when a problem emerges. Sick care involves the medical treatment of a harmful disease, injury, health condition, or symptom.

In contrast to sick care, health care pushes you to act before symptoms appear. By bolstering your immune system with vitamin C, antioxidants, and plenty of water, you take a proactive approach to your health rather than waiting until you experience cold or flu symptoms.

The value of being proactive with your health cannot be emphasized enough. It may seem simpler to wait until a problem emerges and then go to the doctor, but sick care carries more risk and will cost more in the long term.

Consider a nagging old college sports injury. After playing games with your friends over the weekend, you ice it and explain it away as just part of advancing in age. You may think that you can ignore it for several years more, but one day you may find yourself making an appointment with an orthopedic surgeon for surgery. Even with excellent health insurance, the procedure means lost wages, missed social and community events, a temporary loss of mobility, and excruciating pain.

A proactive approach to healthcare understands the significance of dealing with problems like this early on before they become expensive concerns that require ongoing care for months of being unable to do daily activities or even for the rest of one's life. Being more proactive and taking control of your health can be quite empowering, especially if you are feeling victimized by a chronic illness.

Prevent Illness With Acupuncture

There are proven effective strategies to actively safeguard your health and prevent disease. Foremost among them are lifestyle changes involving better nutrition, exercise, stress avoidance, and sufficient sleep. Along with these lifestyle measures, acupuncture is a powerful tool for disease prevention. Your acupuncturist is the health advocate that can help you pursue a proactive course through various phases of your life. Your acupuncturist will not only provide you with customized treatments each time but also guide you with nutrition and herbal supplements that are uniquely suitable for you, your body type, and your needs as they change over time.

As an example, acupuncture has long been used to treat diabetes and its consequences in China. Previous studies suggested that acupuncture treatment might be helpful for diabetes and its consequences (e.g., stomach problems and foot numbness). Acupuncture is now being used more frequently to prevent diabetes. According to research, acupuncture may help prediabetic individuals (those with high blood sugar on the verge of diabetes) with weight loss, lowering of fasting plasma glucose (FPG), 2-hour plasma glucose (2-hPG), and HbA1c levels, as well as a return to normal blood sugar levels (Shi et al., 2018).

Another example is the use of acupuncture in the prevention of sports injuries. It has been demonstrated that acupuncture can effectively prevent sports injuries in professional athletes. This is important because sports injuries can keep athletes from participating in sports activities long term. The greatest enemy of athletes in all sports is muscle damage. For example, in soccer, 20%–40% of all sports-related injuries are muscle-related, primarily affecting the lower limbs.

In a recent study, 54 male athletes from a professional football team were studied for the effect of acupuncture in preventing muscle injuries. The athletes were divided into six groups of nine, with five groups receiving various acupuncture treatments and one group receiving none (the control group). The athletes continued their usual sports routine during the study period. After eight weeks with one acupuncture session per week, only 4 of 45 athletes (9%) receiving acupuncture presented with muscle injuries, while 6 of 9 athletes (67%) not receiving acupuncture had muscle injuries (Dias Junior, 2019).

Consider regular acupuncture treatments as your preventive tune-up. Traditional Chinese Medicine practitioners in ancient times gave everyone routine community care rather than only emergency treatment when someone was ill or hurt. In contrast, the majority of patients today in the U.S. and other Western nations only seek acupuncture treatments when they are ill or in pain.

In the West, our studies have mostly concentrated on acupuncture's potential as a treatment for particular illnesses. For instance, studies have shown that acupuncture can ease psychiatric problems such as post-traumatic stress disorder (PTSD), lessen nausea, and reduce vomiting after chemotherapy. It can also relieve chronic low back pain, tooth pain, migraine headaches, fibromyalgia, and osteoarthritis symptoms.

To keep the focus on health maintenance, Traditional Chinese Medicine practitioners frequently use acupuncture as a form of "tune-up" that is employed as a preventative measure. Such tune-ups are provided by acupuncturists to restore the body's natural homeostasis and to stop minor annoyances from developing into serious issues.

Patients who are experiencing acute ailments can experience positive improvements with acupuncture quite fast, and some of them may stop going for visits. However, the main benefit of acupuncture is the whole-body balance and realignment that can happen once the acute problems have been treated. Many people pay closer attention to the acupuncturist's recommendations for preventive measures, such as lifestyle, nutrition, and, of course, preventive acupuncture treatments, once their first experience with acupuncture proves beneficial.

For example, to help your body adjust to changing environmental circumstances and to strengthen your immune system against external pathogenic influences, it is recommended that you receive preventative acupuncture treatments at least four times a year, once at the start of each season. For patients with chronic diseases, one preventive session per month is suggested once they have recovered following a course of therapies in order to avoid any relapses. To boost protection against pollen in patients with seasonal allergies, it is essential to schedule at least two or three preventive sessions each year before Spring. My patients love their acupuncture tune-ups. Some schedule them at the end of their busy work week to feel refreshed before they start their weekend. One patient often calls his tune-up his staycation. Not many other medical treatments can boast such rewarding and restorative sensations patients feel not just during but also after their "tune-up."

Chapter 4:

Balance and Well-Being—a Holistic Approach

Health is the state of balance, and Traditional Chinese Medicine helps the body restore its balance. When the body is in balance, it naturally regulates the immune system, fights inflammation, viruses, and infections, and normalizes hormones. With this simple approach, Traditional Chinese Medicine safely and effectively addresses many modern-day maladies, such as pain, stress, anxiety, hormonal imbalances, digestive issues, allergies, insomnia, brain fog, and sexual dysfunctions.

Western medicine measures a patient's level of well-being by the absence of symptoms. You are said to be healthy if you don't have any specific symptoms, like a headache or asthma, even though you might not feel "on top of your game." Traditional Chinese Medicine strives to fulfill a higher purpose, realizing that feeling good is more than just the absence of obvious symptoms. We may all feel better than we do now by relaxing and achieving harmony throughout the body.

Achieving Balance

Debbie was a 63-year-old female with a history of cancer. When she first came to me, she was suffering from a nervous breakdown. She had to deal with a lot of stress and grief in her life and presented with chronic fatigue. Vertigo, tinnitus, and joint and low back pain also pestered her. Here is her testimonial after receiving a course in acupuncture: "Just wanted to share: I feel so unexpectedly amazing today—a sense of balance and calm. I slept deeply and felt energized."

Debbie's testimonial beautifully summarizes what we will be discussing in this chapter: the incredible power of acupuncture to give you a sense of well-being, "a sense of balance and calm," as Debbie puts it.

One of the key factors driving patients to acupuncturists in the West over the past several decades has been the improvement in the patient's overall well-being. The holistic care acupuncture patients receive is noticeably different from the therapy they receive from the wide range of specialists they are used to seeing as they visit the various clinics and outpatient sections of our hospitals.

The term "holistic" comes from the Greek word *holos*, meaning "whole," and it refers to treating the patient as a whole rather than only the symptoms isolated from the context of the person experiencing them. In Traditional Chinese Medicine and acupuncture, the focus is on holistic treatment. In addition to the physical symptoms (such as nausea, fever, bloating, or pain), the emotional symptoms (such as stress or anxiety) are also significant because we do not live in a bubble. Our living environment has an impact on our health. Everything affects us, including what we eat, taste, smell, see, and touch. Our health is impacted by anything, from what we read on our phones to what we discuss with our friends.

The idea that the body and mind are interconnected, interact, and influence one another makes Traditional Chinese Medicine so alluring. It acknowledges the significance of the environment, diet, and lifestyle and provides support and guidance in these areas.

From the perspective of Traditional Chinese Medicine, treatment of the physical body affects mental and emotional health, and vice versa, because there is no distinction between them in this system of medicine. Physical problems frequently point us toward an underlying emotional imbalance, which is then treated with the help of acupuncture.

Such emotional releases and balancing might be somewhat surprising when they first occur to a patient. Regardless of the condition for which someone receives treatment, they frequently find acupuncture wonderfully calming. Additionally, most patients note an improvement in their energy levels, sleep quality, and overall sense of well-being.

Traditional Chinese Medicine doesn't separate the mind from the body and doesn't view the body as a sum of disjointed and compartmentalized parts. Furthermore, illness is regarded as the dysfunction of a usually healthy, full-bodied living being due to an imbalance rather than the disease of discrete organs, muscles, joints, or a limb as though they were only gears in a machine.

In the West, many astounding advancements have been made as a result of the perception that the human body is merely a highly developed machine, including the fantastic advances in surgery and pharmacological therapy. But the limitations of this strategy are a big part of why patients today are not completely satisfied with modern treatment and continue to suffer after invasive therapies. It ignores the fact that the human body is more than the sum of its chemistry and mechanics working in concert together and that the mind and emotions have a very strong influence on the body.

When treating a patient, an acupuncturist looks for the "patterns of disharmony" that led to the troubling symptoms. Although acupuncture has recently gained popularity for its effectiveness in treating pain, it has long been used to treat a wide range of illnesses as it fine-tunes the individual. Any symptom may be presented to the acupuncturist by the patient. The acupuncturist's answer is usually the same: Let's pinpoint the pattern of disharmony to identify the root cause before determining the appropriate course of action.

The Traditional Chinese Medicine terms "underlying imbalances" (ben) and "symptoms" (biao) literally mean "root and manifestation," respectively, in Chinese. Traditional Chinese Medicine pays attention to symptoms and works to alleviate them. However, it goes one step further and actively seeks to identify and address the underlying imbalances that lie at the root of symptoms and bring them about. This principle guides the process of diagnosis and treatment in Traditional Chinese Medicine. It is, in fact, the diagnosis approach that dramatically sets Traditional Chinese Medicine apart from its Western counterpart.

That is why, when acupuncture is used to treat these ingrained "imbalances," the patient is frequently surprised to discover that many secondary complaints are also responding in addition to their primary complaint, even some they never thought to disclose to their acupuncturist. It is not unusual to have a patient come in for back pain and notice an improvement in frequent urination, low libido, mood, or their energy level. This is in stark contrast to the results of many modern medications, which often produce secondary complaints due to their side effects.

Many patients seek the help of acupuncturists for advanced health issues that have little to no prospect of improvement. However, even under these circumstances, the patients report that acupuncture treatment has had a significant positive impact on their functional status in a variety of ways. With regular acupuncture treatments, patients frequently experience an increase in vitality, a decrease in discomfort, better sleep, and many other positive changes in their overall health and, as a result, their quality of life. They feel less victimized by a prior diagnosis and regain trust in their body.

Humans are endowed with amazing restorative abilities and resilience. A fever, injury, stress, or emotional anguish may physically or mentally harm an individual. Still, the body, mind, and spirit all have a tendency to return to a balanced state on their own. Homeostasis is the term for this state. The acupuncturist's goal is to support these homeostatic processes. Even if the removal of symptoms is frequently a crucial short-term objective of treatment, it is never the only aim. To determine what level of vitality and health is appropriate given the patient's age, constitution, and circumstances, the practitioner must have a sense of how the patient could be in their restored state of health.

Traditional Chinese Medicine holds that people should balance activity with rest and excitement with reflection. This philosophy of balancing the opposites is known as harmonizing the yin and the yang. Traditional Chinese Medicine uses these terms to explain how opposing natural events balance one another. The ancient Chinese noted that a perpetual transformation of polar opposites occurs in nature. The greatest physicians of ancient China developed a medical system that described how these patterns of change might become imbalanced and result in illness in a person. These ideas convey underlying universal truths. They hold true now as they did more than 2,000 years ago, and they apply equally to patients in the East and the West.

According to the yin/yang theory, all things include variable amounts of yin and yang. They are not substances but represent the opposite poles of the fundamental duality in nature. Chinese ideograms for yin and yang show a hill's gloomy and sunny sides, respectively. The day is yang, and the night is yin. Similar to how day and night perpetually transform into one another in nature, yin and yang are in constant motion.

Yin represents rest, whereas yang represents activity. Yin and yang are continually transforming into one another. The activity must be followed by rest in the same way that summer goes into winter and day into night.

According to the Yellow Emperor's *Classic of Internal Medicine*, one of the acupuncturist's main responsibilities is to closely watch the yin-yang balance and make modifications to achieve equilibrium. Yin corresponds to qualities like cold, dry, and hypoactive, while yang represents factors like hot, wet, and hyperactive. In order to do this, they must assess various factors in their diagnosis of a person's condition. The following simple examples give an idea of how this process is carried out.

Heat or Cold: An acupuncturist can determine a person's yin/yang balance by seeing if that individual is intolerant of cold weather, struggles with hot weather, or can handle either extreme. Various symptoms, such as cold hands and feet, or the opposite—a burning sensation in the hands, feet, or chest—and a preference for hot or iced water are some indications of imbalances in the yin and yang.

Dry or Wet: Dry eyes, dry skin, constipation, a dry cough, and any other dryness-related symptoms are all signs of excessive yang or a deficiency in yin. In contrast, an overabundance of yin or a deficiency in yang in the body can be indicated by symptoms such as swollen ankles, frequent urination, a runny nose, or phlegm.

Hyperactive or Hypoactive: The yang likely outweighs the yin if the person has a predisposition for restlessness, insomnia, quick speech, movement, or emotional volatility. The person's yin is in excess if they have a tendency toward sluggishness, sleepiness, slow speech, and motion, or an emotionless phlegmatic disposition. The body's natural processes sometimes become slow and inert. For instance, a slow heartbeat can signify excess yin, whereas a quick heartbeat could mean excessive yang or insufficient yin.

Based on the patterns of disharmony in yin and yang, an acupuncturist determines if the imbalance is due to an excess in one, a deficiency in the other, or a complex combination of both. As promised, we won't dwell anymore on the yin and yang. Ultimately, achieving a state of equilibrium is the goal of treatments in Traditional Chinese Medicine because when the body is in balance, it naturally heals itself.

Modern medicine has discovered several pervasive control mechanisms in the human body that are strikingly reminiscent of the yin/yang concept. These mechanisms work on the principle of opposing forces and their intricate balance. Research has shown that acupuncture treatment significantly affects and modulates many of these systems.

The billions of cells and various tissues and organs that make up the human body all work together in concert to keep the body healthy. The health of each cell in the body and the body as a whole depends on maintaining a balanced internal environment. The term "homeostasis" refers to all of the various procedures that the body uses to regulate its internal environment.

Internal body variables must be kept within a specific range for the body to function normally; otherwise, disease or illness may develop. When the body is in a homeostasis state, many variables in the body, such as body temperature, blood sugar, blood acidity, water, sodium, calcium, oxygen, blood pressure, heart rate, respiration rate, and all the various hormone levels, continually change in response to internal and external factors to keep the body in a state of balance. When the inner balance is in harmony, we feel energetic, think clearly, have a healthy coping mechanism, sleep well, wake up rested, and feel healthy. The irony lies in the fact that when we feel our best, the last thing on our minds is our body and health. That is exactly when it is important to practice preventive care and be proactive about our health.

A Sense of Well-Being

Acupuncture is powerful in providing you with a wonderful sense of well-being. I experienced this sense of well-being after receiving my very first acupuncture session with my sister. As an acupuncturist, I witness this experience with my patients frequently. A patient writes: "Acupuncture has been my savior for almost two years now! Initially, I came for neck pain—I couldn't turn my head—and ONE visit nearly completely healed it. Since then, my neck and back pain, plus a host of other physical, emotional, and mental ailments, have been tackled! During COVID, regular visits have been the best self-care I could have asked for."

But how do you convey this wonderful experience to someone who has never encountered it and has no clue about it? And how to convince them of its existence in the first place? I can catalog the many health benefits of acupuncture and sing its praises with utmost conviction, but that still cannot give you an idea of what I, and many others, mean by the "wonderful sense of well-being" imparted by acupuncture.

Resorting to research studies and citing scientific literature would not help either. A "wonderful sense of well-being" is an elusive concept, and it would be very difficult to quantify and measure in clinical trials. The problem is compounded by the regrettable fact that acupuncture, as a low-cost treatment, is not the favorite choice for hugely costly trials, even in straightforward topics such as low back pain, let alone for measuring the sense of well-being.

The gentle and soothing practice of acupuncture helps you regain mental and physical balance so you can resume living fully. The physical, emotional, and mental aspects are viewed as interrelated, reflecting what many people see as the relationship between the various aspects of their lives. It is a positive model of health and function, as this patient wrote about her regular treatments: "Acupuncture has become a weekly part of my life. It has allowed me to keep swimming, even though I've been diagnosed with a rotator cuff tear and a bone spur in my right shoulder. I have even been told by my orthopedist that he no longer recommends surgery because my MRIs, only one year apart, are identical—the difference: acupuncture. You don't have to know exactly why you feel acupuncture would help when you walk in. It can help in ways you might not imagine: fatigue, weakness, lethargy, aches, pains, etc. On a regular basis, it has given me strength, both emotionally and physically."

It may be difficult to measure acupuncture's many benefits for promoting well-being in quantitative terms. However, acupuncture affects, in measurable and verifiable ways, many aspects of human physical and mental health that are associated with wellness; physical performance is one example of these factors. Many professional athletes, from Dalvin Cook and Aaron Rodgers to Shaquille O'Neal, Draymond Green, and Olympians DeeDee Trotter and Amy Acuff, turned to acupuncture treatments to enhance recovery and performance. For athletes, acupuncture not only helps prevent injury; it also speeds up recovery and improves performance. Here's what a patient who is an indoor rowing athlete wrote after a qualifying race: "Just wanted to tell you that thanks to you, I had a good race today... I qualified for the world championships... and did much better than last week! Thank you so much for taking good care of me and helping me with this accomplishment. It means a lot to me!"

Chapter 5:

Contemporary Practice of Traditional Chinese Medicine

Traditional Chinese Medicine is highly respected by many medical authorities and overseen by the responsible regulatory bodies at the federal and state levels. It is a recognized form of complementary therapy for various illnesses and health conditions, from chronic low back pain to chemotherapy-induced nausea in people with cancer. The word "complementary" means that acupuncture does not replace conventional medicine in the management of such conditions but helps and complements it. Moreover, people find a strong ally in acupuncture in their daily struggle against insomnia, stress, smoking, obesity, and many other lifestyle problems and in their effort to keep healthy and fit.

Not every illness can be cured by conventional Western medicine. Many people who suffer from anxiety, fibromyalgia, back pain, arthritis, and other chronic ailments turn to complementary therapies rather than potentially dangerous or habit-forming medication to manage their symptoms and reduce the number, frequency, and intensity of flare-ups.

The practice of combining evidence-based complementary therapies with conventional medicine is known as integrative medicine or integrative healthcare. Integrative healthcare aims to develop ways to enhance current treatments rather than to replace conventional medicine. For instance, taking a prescribed medication alone might not be sufficient to help you manage your osteoarthritis. Adding acupuncture to your regimen may give you the edge you need and prevent you from needing a second medicine or more invasive treatments.

Aspects of complementary therapies are becoming increasingly integrated into traditional healthcare as proof of their safety and effectiveness accumulates. A systematic review of medical literature published in December 2021 found that the attitude of healthcare professionals toward acupuncture was positive (Zhang et al., 2023). Today, acupuncture is widely used not only in private clinics but also in hospitals, doctor's offices, and charitable organizations that practice conventional medicine. This acceptance by physicians and healthcare administrators and its great efficacy and safety profile are both contributing factors to acupuncture's rising popularity.

In the late 20th century, Traditional Chinese Medicine and acupuncture spread to many countries. Today, acupuncture is practiced in over one hundred countries, according to the World Health Organization. Acupuncture is used by more than 3 million people in the U.S., but it is even more common elsewhere. One in five people in France, for instance, has used acupuncture.

First, the National Institutes of Health (NIH) acknowledged the effectiveness of acupuncture in treating pain. Later, in 1997, an NIH panel concluded that there was enough evidence from clinical trials to support the benefits of acupuncture and allow its inclusion in conventional medicine. The NIH formally recognized acupuncture for its benefits in treating illnesses like migraines, asthma, stroke recovery, and fibromyalgia, as well as its effectiveness in alleviating nausea brought on by surgery, chemotherapy, or morning sickness. The NIH additionally suggested that medical colleges teach acupuncture (Lu & Lu, 2013).

Since the NIH recognized the benefits of acupuncture, its use has markedly expanded. Today, many hospitals enlist the services of acupuncturists. Over the past decades, acupuncture has spread and gained more acceptance in the U.S. More and more people are incorporating acupuncture as a regular part of their healthcare as the quantity of scientific data supporting it expands. Between the year 2000 and 2010, the number of acupuncture procedures nearly tripled, and nearly 20 million Americans tried acupuncture for various conditions. However, that is still less than 10% of the population; over 90% of Americans have not experienced acupuncture and its many benefits.

Numerous studies have been done in the U.S. and other countries to solve acupuncture's mysteries. Today, there is a wealth of information in the scientific literature on the subject. The findings show that acupuncture stimulation results in the release of endorphins, serotonin, enkephalins, adenosine, gamma-aminobutyric acid (GABA), a major inhibitory neurotransmitter of the brain, norepinephrine, and dopamine (Lin et al., 2012). These changes contribute to explaining the acupuncture effects in biomedical and pharmacological terms in a manner acceptable to the Western medical establishment.

At the same time, at the international level, the World Health Organization (WHO) published a list of conditions it found to be successfully managed by acupuncture in 2003 after conducting a literature study (The World Health Organization, 2003). This list was expanded to include 117 diseases in 2017 by the Acupuncture Evidence Project, supported by the Australian Acupuncture and Chinese Medicine Association (AACMA) (The Acupuncture Evidence Project, 2017).

National Center for Complementary and Integrative Health (NCCIH)

The Office of Alternative Medicine, now known as the National Center for Complementary and Integrative Health (NCCIH), was established by a resolution of the U.S. Congress in 1991, further strengthening the use of acupuncture and other complementary medicines. The NCCIH is the main organization in the federal government that conducts scientific research on alternative and complementary health treatments, including Traditional Chinese Medicine and acupuncture. It conducts research, funds external research, and spreads information about complementary health methods and products (The National Center for Complementary and Integrative Health, 2023).

The goal of NCCIH is to use rigorous scientific research to find out about the scientific basis, usefulness, and safety of complementary and integrative health therapies, as well as how they may improve health and health care. The NCCIH funds various studies to better understand how the body reacts to acupuncture, how acupuncture might work, and how well it works for different types of pain and other illnesses. Recent studies funded by NCCIH include examining the possibility of acupuncture use in medical emergency rooms. Another study aims to determine whether combining acupuncture with transcranial direct current stimulation can improve the treatment of chronic low back pain. A third study investigates an acupuncture-based portable nerve stimulation therapy for anxiety disorders.

The NCCIH is also currently supporting a new funding initiative to create and upkeep a searchable, open-access database and repository for commonly used acupuncture points in the body, or acupoints, along with their anatomical and physiological significance as well as other relevant parameters. The finished database will categorize and explain the available information regarding the anatomical locations and characteristics of the acupoints.

Rigorous Traditional Chinese Medical Training and Licensing

State licensing laws can differ, but there are a few standards that are universal (National Certification Commission for Acupuncture and Oriental Medicine, 2020). A master's degree is first required for acupuncturists in order to practice. They typically have to pass exams to demonstrate their expertise beyond their degree. Generally speaking, acupuncturists must pass exams from the National Certification Commission for Acupuncture and Oriental Medicine (NCCAOM), but certain States, such as California, require licensing through the State's acupuncture board directly.

Traditional Chinese Medicine schools and colleges are regulated by the Accreditation Commission for Acupuncture and Herbal Medicine (ACAHM), an agency recognized by the U.S. Department of Education. The schools offer master's and doctoral programs as well as continuing education courses approved by the State and National regulating bodies. The master's program is over 3200 hours of classroom and clinical training, which takes about four years to complete full-time.

Upon successful completion of the master's program, qualified candidates can apply to sit for examination through the State or National boards that grant licensure to practice Traditional Chinese Medicine within their State. Having earned my Electrical Engineering Bachelor's of Science and Operations Research Master's of Science degrees years prior to completing my Traditional Chinese Medicine master's program, I can attest firsthand that the curriculum at Emperor's College and passing the California Acupuncture Board's licensing requirements were extremely rigorous and required full commitment and dedication.

Depending on their State, acupuncturists must pass specific exams and successfully complete the licensing agency's requirements prior to receiving their license to practice medicine. Most States require NCCAOM certification which grants the designations Dipl. Ac., for Diplomate of Acupuncture, Dipl. C.H. for Diplomate of Chinese Herbology, or Dipl. O.M. for Diplomate of Oriental Medicine, a combination of both acupuncture and herbology certificates. Acupuncture with Point Location, Foundations of Oriental Medicine, Biomedicine, and Chinese Herbology are the four exams offered by the NCCAOM for certification. "Acupuncture with Point Location" includes actions, indications, cautions, and contraindications in addition to anatomical point locations for over 400 acupuncture points. "Biomedicine" includes anatomy, physiology, pathology, pathophysiology, pharmacology, and high-level laboratory and medical imaging knowledge. The "Foundations of Oriental Medicine" covers theory, examination, analysis, and differential diagnosis based on Traditional Chinese Medicine theories, treatment strategies, and principles. The "Chinese Herbology" examination covers the detailed properties, actions, indications, contraindications, and pharmaceutical interactions of single herbs and herbal formulas. States that deviate from NCCAOM examination and licensing requirements have similarly extensive or stringent licensing requirements. The designation L.Ac. stands for Licensed Acupuncturist and is used by some States, such as California, in lieu of the NCCAOM designations.

Once licensed by the Board, practitioners must maintain their license in good standing and keep it active by completing a certain number of approved continuing education credits regularly. In the State of California, where I practice, the renewal requirement is 50 qualified continuing education hours every two years. That requirement is 60 qualified continuing education hours every four years for NCCAOM recertification.

The NCCAOM's Code of Ethics serves as the foundation for its dedication to ethical business conduct and professional behavior. As a requirement for NCCAOM certification and certification maintenance, every acupuncturist receiving NCCAOM certification swears to follow the NCCAOM Code of Ethics norms and guidelines.

Making decisions about your health care, including whether or not to choose complementary health methods, is important. It is crucial to take control of your health by making informed decisions. When seeking a licensed acupuncturist, ask your healthcare provider and those you trust within your community for recommendations. Often, you will find people who highly recommend their acupuncturist as they develop a strong rapport and share their physical, mental, and emotional concerns with their practitioner.

While I highly, strongly, and enthusiastically recommend acupuncture to everyone, I also recognize that it is a complementary approach and urge you to continue seeing your general practitioner for routine and annual check-ups. Ideally, both systems of medicine may be considered complementary, as they truly complement one another. When the two systems are combined, they provide the utmost and most comprehensive care for your health and vitality.

Chapter 6:

Traditional Chinese Medicine Unplugged

Traditional Chinese medicine revolves around a set of unifying principles, but it has various treatment modalities at its disposal—these range from physical interventions like acupuncture and acupressure to herbal remedies and lifestyle counseling. The most important underlying component of Traditional Chinese Medicine, however, is the diagnosis of the root cause according to patterns of disharmony. This means that two individuals with the same Western diagnosis, such as migraine headache, are not given the same treatment as they may have very different root causes for their similar symptoms.

Once the practitioner has concluded a diagnosis according to the pattern differentiation, one or more of the appropriate treatment modalities may be chosen based on the patient's preference and the practitioner's recommendation. In this chapter, we review the various forms of treatments offered under the umbrella of Traditional Chinese medicine at a high level.

Acupuncture

Acupuncture is one of the most recognized and intriguing principal forms of treatment utilized in Traditional Chinese medicine. The treatment consists of inserting needles as thin as a human hair into specific spots on the body to promote balance and healing. Manual manipulation or stimulation with low-level electrical currents may be applied to the needles (electroacupuncture).

According to Traditional Chinese medicine, the key to good health is maintaining a delicate balance within the body. Chinese medicine places a significant emphasis on the concept of qi (pronounced chi), which refers to the vital force that controls all of the processes that occur within the body. Qi travels within the body through channels known as meridians. These energy pathways, through which the qi flows, are accessible through the hundreds of acupuncture points that are spread throughout the body. A disruption or obstruction in the flow of qi can put a person at risk of developing a disease. The energy flow can be restored to its previous state of equilibrium by inserting needles into these sites in the appropriate combinations.

The concept of Qi in Western medicine is not well understood and explained. The meridians and qi are ambiguous as they are not physical and tangible entities and do not fully correspond to the nervous, lymphatic, or vascular systems. Imagine the meridians as invisible electrical conduits hidden in the walls of your house; the acupuncture points are the outlets that let you tap into that electrical system when you plug in your electronic device. How is it that we cannot see these meridians? Same as wireless and cellular technology. We are surrounded by the electromagnetic fields of cellular networks and our Wi-Fi network. Although invisible, this web of connectivity helps us communicate through devices unimaginable just decades ago. The concept of a life force, qi, energy, or current flowing through invisible meridians is no longer hard to imagine and accept if we are open to thinking outside the box regarding our bodies. We are composed of living cells, and living cells produce electromagnetic fields. The meridians in our body are fields of electromagnetic energy similar to cellular networks, wireless communication, the world wide web, and the invisible orbits in the cosmos.

Acupuncture is used to treat pain and various illnesses. Some researchers think the needles induce the body to produce endorphins, which are the body's natural painkillers. They also think that the needles may increase blood flow and alter brain activity to good effect.

It has been demonstrated that stimulating specific acupuncture sites impacts brain regions that are known to lessen sensitivity to pain and stress while also encouraging relaxation. Neurological system stimulation by acupuncture triggers the release of neurochemical messenger molecules. The resulting biochemical alterations impact the body's inner balance, enhancing physical and mental health.

Acupuncture switches your sympathetic nervous system off and removes you from "fight-or-flight" mode. At the same time, it relaxes you by turning on your parasympathetic nervous system. This system is normally activated when you eat or take a break. Acupuncture stops the cycle of stress that seems to never end, so you can unwind and recover from the continuous state of "fight-or-flight."

Acupuncture calms you down. Many patients doze off while receiving treatment. They nap in the middle of the session and wake up feeling refreshed, which is why some refer to their acupuncture treatment as nap-time or acu-nap.

Additionally, acupuncture makes you feel happy. Studies have revealed that when you undergo acupuncture, your body releases the "feel-good" hormone, serotonin. You essentially get the feeling of excitement or "runner's high."

Acupuncture alters the brain's mood chemistry to help fight off negative emotions by regulating levels of neurotransmitters and hormones such as endorphin, serotonin, noradrenaline, dopamine, GABA, neuropeptide Y, and ACTH. By boosting endorphin levels and decreasing serotonin levels, acupuncture can change the brain's chemicals to improve mood and lessen the effects of depressive states (Lin et al., 2012).

While acupuncture is commonly referred to as inserting needles in specific acupuncture points, musculoskeletal issues often require the placement of needles in areas of the muscles that do not correspond to acupuncture points. This is done to release trigger points, alleviate pain, and relieve spasms and knots at the site of the needle. Acupuncturists refer to these points as ah-shi points, which literally means tender-points or ouch-points. Non-acupuncturist healthcare practitioners may receive training to practice a technique called "Dry Needling," which treats musculoskeletal pain using acupuncture needles similar to the treatment of ah-shi points by acupuncturists.

Acupressure is when acupuncture points are used without the insertion of acupuncture needles. The practice of acupressure is performed at the same places along the energy channels as acupuncture but without the use of needles. By gently stimulating these points, qi and blood flow are restored. Acupressure involves gentle but firm stimulation of acupuncture points using fingers, thumbs, and elbows. Acupressure may be combined with acupuncture and is often used for patients with a weaker constitution who respond best to less stimulation.

Herbal Medicine

Herbal medicine, or herbology, is another major component of Traditional Chinese Medicine. In Traditional Chinese Medicine, herbs are prescribed to treat patterns of disharmony, similar to acupuncture. Unlike in Western herbal medicine, herbs are rarely used singly in this system of medicine. In Traditional Chinese Medicine, most prescriptions contain multiple herbs, referred to as a formula, that together have a synergistic effect. The combination of herbs is chosen for each patient based on their unique diagnosis.

Traditional Chinese herbs are safe when properly sourced and given by a properly trained and licensed practitioner. Adverse effects are rare with Chinese herbal therapy, but they can happen with any type of medicine.

Herbal remedies are prescribed in raw or powdered forms. Powdered herbs are often diluted in water as reconstructed tea for consumption. Alternatively, they sometimes come in the form of capsules or tablets. If you are prescribed raw herbs, the practitioner will provide you with specific instructions on how to boil them to make a tea that you can drink multiple times a day.

Cupping Therapy

Cupping therapy is another traditional Chinese medicine treatment that is often practiced in conjunction with acupuncture. In cupping, hot glass or plastic cups are vacuum-pumped over a part of the body, such as the legs or the back, to remove obstructions and promote the flow of qi and blood. Cupping can loosen up tense muscles, promote healing, and lessen discomfort. Cupping is not limited to Traditional Chinese Medicine and has been a common practice in the Mediterranean, Middle East, and Russia for a long time.

Many people compare the sensation of cupping to a deep massage. Cupping relieves congestion, chronic tension, and acute muscle spasms. Cupping promotes circulation and helps your body detoxify naturally. The fresh blood supply restored to the area helps with regeneration and nourishes the tissue. You may get cupping as a standalone treatment, or your practitioner may add it to your acupuncture session if needed. Patients often feel immediate relief after cupping: "I had a cupping session done, and I felt all the pain being lifted off my body in just one session. I walked to the car as light as a feather. This was just what I needed for my ongoing shoulder and neck pain. I can't wait to go back!"

For many people, the main concern about cupping is that it may cause bruising. It is true; cupping may result in bruising because it vacuums old stagnant blood, lymph, and body fluids out of the tissue, bringing them to the skin's surface, which is the body's biggest detox organ. This allows fresh blood supply to the tissue and promotes faster healing and recovery. Bruises typically resolve within 3–5 days.

Chronic neck, shoulder, and back pain can be successfully treated by cupping. It is an excellent treatment for athletes wanting to recover faster from their training and anyone with recent physical trauma, such as a car accident. Cupping helps open skin pores; therefore, it is best to keep extra warm after the treatment. It is recommended to have warm clothing and a scarf for post-treatment and avoid exposure to cold drafts following your appointment.

Gua Sha

Gua sha promotes the flow of the essential elements qi and blood, much like cupping. The practitioner will use a scraping or pressing technique to make petechiae or "sha" appear on the skin while using lubricating oil and a gua sha tool. The sha that appears indicates the release of stagnated blood and body fluids in the tissue due to trauma or muscle spasm. The sha markings disappear over time and may last up to a week.

Gua sha helps loosen the muscles and restore blood flow in the area. It aids in relaxing the fascia, mobilizing soft tissue, and is excellent at reducing scars. It is also referred to as the "Graston Technique" when utilized by non-acupuncturist health care practitioners. Like cupping, gua sha opens up skin pores; hence, it is important to keep warm after the treatment and avoid drafts.

Moxibustion

The traditional Chinese herb known as moxa is used frequently in a technique called moxibustion. "Moxa" is made up of dried leaves of the mugwort plant and is known for its capacity to promote warmth and blood flow.

Moxibustion can be used in conjunction with acupuncture or alone. The moxa is frequently burned on or close to the needle's handle when used with acupuncture to deliver warmth to the point for additional stimulation. It can also be applied directly to the skin using a medium such as a slice of ginger or held near the skin using a moxa stick which looks similar to a cigar. Patients may also use the moxa stick at home on certain acupuncture points as prescribed by their practitioner.

Tui Na

Using many of the same acupuncture concepts, tui na is a form of manual bodywork that stimulates the flow of qi to produce balance and harmony within the body. The words *tui*, which means "to push," and *na*, which means "to lift and squeeze," are the origin of the term. The practitioner applies traction, range-of-motion, and acupressure point stimulation.

Techniques might be very soft or quite solid. Practitioners utilize pressure and oscillation techniques with varying speeds and forces during a session. Tui na massage can be used as an energizing therapy or a more powerful deep-tissue massage.

In contrast to Western massage techniques, tui na works with the body on a more profound energy level, going beyond the muscles, bones, and joints. The practitioner may use manipulation techniques to press, rub, knead, roll, and brush the spaces between the joints, called the eight gates, to unlock the body's defensive qi and get the energy going. During a session of tui na, the practitioner uses their hands to detect the client's energy and change how that energy is distributed and flows.

Tai Chi and Qigong

Tai chi and qigong are movement exercises done in a gentle, deliberate manner. They are meant to strengthen and balance the body while calming the mind. In tai chi, your entire body moves as a single unit, and balance in motion is emphasized. It consists of a series of flowing motions that target the entire body. On the other hand, qigong is performed as a single movement that is done repeatedly as a form of healing therapy. For example, the practitioner may concentrate on one qigong move that helps open the lungs. Both tai chi and qigong are extremely relaxing and harmonizing for the body and mind.

Nutritional Coaching

In contrast to Western medicine, Traditional Chinese Medicine places major emphasis on nutrition, not just to nourish but to treat the body. Traditional Chinese Medicine categorizes foods into five natures: cold, cool, neutral, warm, and hot. The character of food is determined by how it affects a person's body after eating, not by how hot or cold it is to touch. A person's body is impacted when they consistently eat one type of food, which leads to a state of imbalance. Maintaining our body's 'neutrality' and balance is at the heart of Traditional Chinese Medicine.

There's more to the taste than meets the tongue. Traditional Chinese Medicine further categorizes foods into five categories: sour, bitter, sweet, spicy, and salty. These, however, are more than just senses for our taste buds. According to Traditional Chinese Medicine, each flavor of food sends nutrition to the corresponding organs: salt enters the kidneys and can drain, purge, and soften material; bitter food enters the heart and small intestine; it helps to cool heat and dry any dampness; spicy food enters the lungs and large intestine; it helps to stimulate appetite and warm the body; and sweet food enters the stomach and spleen; it helps to moisten the body.

In Traditional Chinese Medicine, no one size fits everyone. The preceding points do not imply that we need to consume a fixed food combination to stay healthy. People have various body constitutions, just like we all have different personalities. And just as you cannot interact with everyone in the same manner, neither can you nourish your body in the same way all the time. The design of your body, the time of year, where you live, and your state of health all impact the foods you choose to eat. Age and sex may also affect the physical condition. In other words, Chinese medical professionals customize their recommendations according to an individual's constitution and condition at the given time.

Lifestyle Coaching

Following a holistic approach, Traditional Chinese Medicine does not limit itself to therapeutic interventions and nutritional coaching. It recognizes the crucial role of various aspects of lifestyle, from exercise habits to sex to the value of friendship and social relationships, on health and well-being. Once again, the goal of Traditional Chinese Medicine is to restore and maintain balance, offering pearls of wisdom to achieve this in all aspects of one's life.

A positive outcome of the COVID-19 pandemic was enabling acupuncturists to practice telehealth. The success of telehealth in this medicine is a testament to the value of Traditional Chinese medicine's lifestyle coaching, along with self-acupressure and nutrition therapy. During the pandemic, the following patient suffering from back pain shared about her telehealth experience: "Thank you for my COVID-times video acupuncture session. It was so much better than I expected it would be to see you 'virtually' instead of in person. I know it would be even better to actually get the needles and your healing touch in person... But I feel MUCH less pain today than I did yesterday."

Chapter 7:

What to Expect in Your Acupuncture Session

People new to acupuncture often have legitimate questions and concerns about this form of therapy. They may want to know how this new experience will unfold. In this chapter, we walk through the stages of typical acupuncture treatment—before, during, and after the treatment—to allay these concerns and prepare you to get the most out of your visit and enjoy your treatment.

Before You Arrive

You may receive a health history questionnaire from your acupuncturist prior to your appointment. It is often very detailed and will ask for information seemingly not relevant to your chief complaint. Take time to complete this form in its entirety. As mentioned throughout this book, Traditional Chinese Medicine identifies and treats the root causes of your symptoms. The questionnaires are often meticulously designed by your practitioner to help with identifying patterns of disharmony and honing in on the root cause. Taking some time to complete the form in advance helps you get the most out of your initial visit. Feel free to call and ask your acupuncturist any questions you may have before your appointment.

It is best to consume a small meal a few hours before your visit. Acupuncture is not administered to those who are fasting. At the same time, don't overindulge or consume something that will upset your stomach (for example, rich, greasy, fried, or extremely spicy foods).

Overeating raises the likelihood of experiencing nausea. On the day of your treatment, abstain from alcohol. Intoxicated people are not treated with acupuncture.

Often, you may receive your acupuncture treatment without having to disrobe. The limbs below the knees and elbows are where the majority of the most commonly used acupuncture points are found. Dress comfortably in loose-fitting clothing so that you can roll up your clothing to above your elbows and knees without restricting your circulation while staying warm during the treatment. As the body starts the healing process, it promotes blood flow to the sites that need repair, and as a result, it is not unusual to feel cold during the treatment. Acupuncturists often have heat lamps or heated tables to keep the patient comfortable during the treatment.

It is recommended that you do not scrape or brush your tongue on the day of the treatment. During the examination, your acupuncturist will ask to see your tongue, and the tongue's coat reveals important information about your health.

Bring a list of all the drugs you are currently taking, including prescriptions, over-the-counter medicine, herbal remedies, and supplements. Bring any laboratory or medical results that are pertinent to your condition.

During Your Session

An extensive evaluation of your chief complaint while reviewing your health history is a thorough process and may take up most of your first appointment.

The acupuncturist will ask you about topics throughout the assessment that you don't think to have anything to do with your primary complaints, such as your diet, cravings, emotions, sleeping habits, bowel movements, and digestion patterns. The collection of symptoms and indicators you are exhibiting come together to reveal patterns of imbalance that indicate the underlying cause of your complaint.

Your practitioner will ask to see your tongue, as it reveals much information about your overall health, such as digestion, circulation, metabolism, energy level, hot/cold nature, and even emotional wellness. I often say a tongue doesn't lie!

Next, your practitioner will take your pulse on both wrists. Pulse diagnosis, similar to tongue diagnosis, provides additional information that further supports narrowing down the root cause. When taking the pulse, the practitioner feels for the quality of the pulse as it resonates under slight pressure, such as being slippery like a string of pearls or wiry like a guitar string. Other qualities, such as the depth at which the pulse is felt the strongest and the relevant pulsation speed, reveal further diagnostic information to your acupuncturist.

Once a diagnosis is reached, your treatment begins. Acupuncture points will be chosen based on the information gathered, the assessment, and the examination. Your practitioner will place the needles and then allow you to rest for about 30 minutes, at which point the needles will be removed. During the treatment, you may feel nothing happening, or you may feel sleepy or experience a heavy sensation, pulsation, or tingling in your arms, legs, or other parts of the body. These sensations may be felt at the site of the needles or along the meridians that your acupuncture points are stimulating. Acupuncturists take extra care to ensure their patients are at ease during the treatment so they can unwind while the needles are in. Many patients doze off during acupuncture. Your session may also involve other therapies such as cupping or gua sha, herbal prescriptions, and dietary and lifestyle recommendations.

After Your Session

After an acupuncture treatment, it is typical to experience extreme calmness and relaxation.

To get the most out of your treatments, it is best to rest and avoid scheduling any activities after your acupuncture session. The treatment is not finished once your session is over; rather, it only serves to initiate or reinforce a longer-term healing process.

Avoid cold drafts and dress warmly if your treatment includes gua sha or cupping.

It is recommended not to consume alcohol just after receiving treatment. Immediately following a treatment, the body may be more sensitive to stimulants due to the detoxifying nature of acupuncture.

Individual treatment results vary. Your relief might start right away, take a little while to come on, or possibly take one to three days. The first treatment may only provide temporary relief, but subsequent treatments reinforce the previous treatment, and the relief will increasingly last longer. Ideally, the treatments are scheduled in such a way that the results last until your next appointment.

Although uncommon, mild side effects can include feeling lightheaded, dizzy, sleepy, or nauseated. You may also experience bruising at the site of the needles or feel some lingering muscle aches. Any of these symptoms should pass quickly. Staying hydrated and getting rest after your treatment will also help reduce these symptoms. At your subsequent visit, talk about your experience with your acupuncturist.

Rarely, following a treatment, one's initial symptoms could momentarily worsen or "flare up." Other names for this include a healing crisis or a healing event. A healing crisis may indicate the body is detoxifying or that it is fighting something, such as a virus. In this case, you could feel sleepy after therapy because your body is using all of its resources to heal, combat a virus, or fight an infection. Flare-ups typically occur later in the day of your treatment and might last anywhere from a few hours to days. Your signs and symptoms should start to get better after a flare-up. Acupuncture does not, over time, worsen any symptoms.

How soon can you anticipate feeling better? Generally speaking, if the problem is acute, an improvement could be noticed after a few or even only one treatment. For chronic illnesses, several treatments over time will be needed to help the condition get better and restore the body's balance.

The best course of action for a disease is to start treatment as soon as feasible. The earlier you seek care, the easier it is to treat the condition and slow down or stop its progression. For lasting results, it is important to complete the recommended course of treatment once you start the healing process. Results improve with consistency.

Acupuncture's results are cumulative and accrue over time. Once your initial symptoms resolve, a few more treatments might be suggested to reinforce the results. This is referred to as "solidifying the constitution" in Traditional Chinese Medicine. The objective is to fortify your body further so the ailment won't return.

The frequency of treatments is determined by the condition and the individual's response. Since the effects of acupuncture are cumulative and develop over time as the body regains its balance, the duration between treatments will increase. At some point, you will reach a maintenance phase, choose to go for treatments only when you feel you need a tune-up or miss that blissful post-acupuncture feeling.

Chapter 8:

A Complementary Treatment for Modern-Day Conditions

Traditional Chinese Medicine is a powerful tool and a potent complementary treatment for fighting a wide range of physical and emotional disorders, diseases, and pain. In this final chapter, let us briefly review the scientific evidence for the efficacy of acupuncture against some of the most commonly treated conditions.

Arthritis—Osteoarthritis

Osteoarthritis is the most prevalent kind of arthritis. Usually, it progresses with advancing age. Any joint can be affected, but the knees, hips, hands, lower back, and neck are where most patients experience pain. As the joint loses cartilage with wear and tear, the bone grows to try and repair the damage. But instead of improving things, the bone grows atypically and exacerbates the situation. The bone changes may cause discomfort and instability in the joint. This may impact your physical well-being or capacity to move the affected joint.

Acupuncture can be beneficial for patients with osteoarthritis. According to a Cochrane evaluation studying the impact of acupuncture on osteoarthritis, the treatment may have a small positive effect on patients' pain and physical function (Manheimer et al., 2010). The American College of Rheumatology, a professional organization for doctors specializing in arthritis, approves acupuncture as a complementary treatment for hand, knee, and hip pain. The strongest data points to its potential benefit for knees (Hochberg et al., 2012).

Acupuncture may reduce arthritis pain by altering the pain signals your brain receives from damaged tissues and by promoting the production of your body's natural painkillers (endorphins and enkephalin). When you first start treatment, this pain alleviation might only last a short while, but continued treatment (often once per week for six or more weeks) might produce long-term improvement, frequently lasting for many months. If the discomfort returns, more acupuncture may help. Acupuncture can be helpful at practically any stage of arthritis and may potentially slow the progression of the wear and tear; however, there is no scientific evidence that it can reverse the tissue damage already done.

Autoimmune Disease: Rheumatoid Arthritis

The chronic inflammatory disease rheumatoid arthritis (RA) affects the entire body, particularly the joints. It is an autoimmune illness, which means that instead of defending the body against infections, the immune system incorrectly starts to attack healthy tissue. Pain in the joints is one of the most prevalent signs of RA.

Acupuncture treatment may be appealing to those with painful diseases, such as joint pain from RA. Acupuncture cannot cure rheumatoid arthritis but can help with joint pain and reduce flare-up frequency. It is a pain-relieving technique with few side effects that can be used in conjunction with prescription therapy. A systematic review of the efficacy of acupuncture on rheumatoid arthritis assessed 43 studies and concluded that acupuncture is beneficial in the treatment of rheumatoid arthritis without adverse effects and can improve patients' function and quality of life (Chou & Chu, 2018).

Autoimmune Disease: Psoriasis and Psoriatic Arthritis

Psoriasis is an autoimmune disease that results in red or purple scaly skin areas that can peel, itch, and bleed. Joint pain, edema, and stiffness can be brought on by psoriatic arthritis, which affects some people with psoriasis. Treatments for these problems include utilizing skin creams to assist in controlling peeling and scale buildup, immune system reaction control medications, and anti-inflammatory medications.

Psoriasis can be treated with acupuncture in a number of ways. It works well to reduce stress, and stress is a frequent cause of psoriasis flare-ups. Additionally, it can lessen pain, particularly in instances of psoriatic arthritis. A systematic review of 13 clinical trials with 1,060 participants examined the efficacy of acupuncture on psoriasis. The authors came to the conclusion that acupuncture-related methods could be utilized as a complementary treatment for the illness (Yeh et al., 2017).

Headaches and Migraines

If you are one of the millions of individuals who have migraines or tension headaches, you surely already know that resting and over-the-counter medication don't always work. For this reason, alternative therapies, particularly acupuncture, are becoming more popular. Research evidence and plenty of patient testimonials point to the efficacy of acupuncture in this regard.

In 2020, researchers from several U.S. medical schools published a paper giving an overview of numerous systematic reviews on the subject of acupuncture in migraines, distilling the results of many clinical studies. They stated that although medication therapy is the main treatment for migraines, acupuncture is receiving more recognition as a practical complement to the care of migraine patients because of its demonstrable effects on the length and frequency of migraine attacks. According to the paper's authors, numerous studies indicate that acupuncture is a secure, practical, and accessible alternative therapy that may aid people with migraine (Urits et al., 2020).

A recent study enrolled 147 people with migraines from 7 hospitals to see how acupuncture affected them. All of the patients had never had acupuncture before, and they were told not to begin any new treatments or take any painkillers during the trial. Patients were randomly divided into three groups and given eight weeks of standard therapy, which included lifestyle and self-management counseling, 20 sessions of acupuncture, or 20 sessions of sham acupuncture. According to the findings, acupuncture treatment significantly reduced the number of migraine days and migraine attacks more than sham acupuncture or standard medical care (Xu et al., 2020).

Low Back Pain

Low back pain is one of the most common causes of seeking medical attention. It is also one of the top reasons for acupuncture use. Often, treatment will include physical manipulation in addition to acupuncture. Acute low back pain may be resolved in as little as one session. Here's what a new patient wrote about her treatment for low back pain: "I just wanted to say that I absolutely loved my acupuncture/cupping experience. I had so much energy, and my back pain disappeared!"

Research shows that acupuncture can be an effective treatment for low back pain. A systematic review assessed clinical studies involving 17,922 patients and concluded that acupuncture is a viable alternative for referral since it effectively treats chronic pain (Vickers et al., 2012).

Sciatica

The sciatic nerve originates from the spine in the low back. After passing through the hips, it descends the leg all the way down to the heel of the foot. Compression of the sciatic nerve causes sciatica, which produces low back pain radiating to the legs. Spinal stenosis or disc issues, such as degeneration and herniation, are frequent causes of this condition. Low back pain, tingling or numbness that travels down the leg to the foot, and weakness in the affected areas are sciatica symptoms.

Sciatica can be effectively treated with acupuncture without the negative effects of over-the-counter painkillers such as non-steroidal anti-inflammatory drugs (NSAIDs) and muscle relaxants. Acupuncture can help reduce the dosage and adverse effects of drugs that are prescribed for sciatica by enhancing their effectiveness. In one systematic review of acupuncture use for sciatica, 11 studies with 962 patients were evaluated. It was found that acupuncture treated sciatica symptoms more effectively than NSAIDs (Qin et al., 2015).

Another patient, a medical doctor trying acupuncture for the first time, wrote this about her experience with acupuncture for sciatica pain: "My patients and I often suffer chronic pain that allopathic medicine relieves poorly. While on the cruise, the introductory consultation persuaded me to try acupuncture. I can recommend this treatment with confidence. I am a long-distance runner in my late 50s. When I over-exercise or even consistently push myself over several weeks, I begin experiencing an ache in my hips and buttocks, mostly sciatic pain. Acupuncture relieved this pain; whether it will persist after acute treatment remains to be seen; however, nothing else has worked so well. In addition, after an hour of relaxing with the needles in, I felt reenergized, as if I were walking taller. Also, I have never felt so free of tension as during the treatment."

Sprains and Strains

Any strain, which is a stretch or tear in a muscle or its tendon, or sprain, which is a stretch or tear in a bone ligament, manifests in its first or acute stage with varied degrees of pain, swelling, and bruising. The muscles around the trauma site tense to protect the damaged location, causing the area to become stiff. This defensive behavior prevents robust blood flow to the area, even though the blood contains the necessary healing ingredients.

Treatment for the pain and inflammation must start right away. The immediate treatment for these types of injuries consists of Rest, Ice, Compression, and Elevation, or RICE for short. The best place to start is by relieving pressure on the injured joint, elevating it, and using ice to reduce swelling and inflammation over the initial 48 to 72 hours to avoid causing tissue injury. It's crucial to reduce swelling; however, using ice for an extended period of time may limit movement and actually impede the healing process. The vascular constriction caused by the cold limits blood flow to the location. It may be pleasant because ice numbs the area temporarily. However, the injured area needs to receive fresh, oxygenated blood and nutrients to heal.

Treatment with acupuncture is helpful for injuries that produce a lot of swelling after emergency management. In fact, it is one of the best methods for improving blood flow in cases of acute ankle sprains and other sprains or strains. This helps bring tissue-healing oxygen and nutrients to the injured area. Acupuncture can also decrease muscle tension and provide pain relief. The end result is that you will recover more quickly from the injury and need fewer rest days.

Here's what one massage therapist shared about her treatments for sprains and strains: "I have had great results each time I have been treated with acupuncture. The first time was for a strained and inflamed shoulder, and the second was for a dislocated and badly sprained index finger. The results were amazing, and the inflammation was reduced almost immediately, and in the case of my shoulder, gone completely within 24 hours, and I was pain-free!"

Neuropathy

Damage to the nerves that transmit signals between the brain, spinal cord, and the rest of the body results in peripheral neuropathy. Such an injury might result in numbness, weakness, and discomfort in the hands, legs, or feet. Not every patient with neuropathy experiences the same symptoms since there are several forms of this condition. The majority of them, however, report changes in their mobility, excessive sensitivity to touch, weakened muscles, heat intolerance, and acute pain that keep them from carrying out daily tasks. Diabetes, chemotherapy side effects, exposure to chemicals, and other medical conditions are some of the significant risk factors that might cause neuropathy.

People with neuropathy frequently use acupuncture to treat their numbness, tingling, pain, and discomfort. Acupuncture also increases blood flow to repair damaged nerves, whether it is due to a chronic disease such as diabetes or a repetitive strain injury, as in this musician's case: "I was experiencing numbness in my left hand and arm from playing the acoustic bass. I received acupuncture treatments, and after three visits, my arm was completely healed. I had feeling back in my hand, and my bass playing improved. I highly recommend acupuncture to anyone—it helped me immensely!"

In 2017, Alexandra Dimitrova published an important paper describing a series of cases where people with peripheral neuropathy had received acupuncture. All patients reported improvements in their symptoms (Dimitrova, 2017).

Dentistry Pain

Dental work discomfort frequently demands the use of anesthetics, while dental surgery postoperative pain is typically managed with over-the-counter pain relievers or opioid painkillers. Acupuncture provides an alternative method of treating dental pain; it also helps many people who feel dental anxiety when having dental work done. The use of acupuncture as an analgesic for postoperative dental pain was one of the first medical applications of acupuncture recognized by the NIH (NIH Consensus Conference, 1998).

In recent years, a controlled study randomly assigned 60 patients to an acupuncture group and a drug group receiving conventional local anesthesia before tooth extraction. According to the findings, acupuncture anesthesia for tooth extraction had the same impact as anesthetic drugs. Its analgesia was complete, with stabilized vital signs and fewer side effects (Pan et al., 2017).

Adrenal Fatigue

Adrenal fatigue is not a recognized medical term; rather, it is a name used to describe a group of general symptoms, such as body aches, fatigue, nervousness, disturbed sleep, and digestive issues. These symptoms may be brought on by the adrenal glands not functioning properly in the presence of prolonged mental, emotional, or physical stress. According to Western medicine, stress impacts the hypothalamic-pituitary-adrenal (HPA) axis, which interferes with the body's ability to maintain homeostasis and results in various disabling symptoms.

Adrenal fatigue may be a mild form of chronic stress-related adrenal insufficiency. According to certain studies, fibromyalgia and hypothyroidism may also have a relationship with adrenal fatigue.

Some signs of adrenal fatigue include:

- being emotionally and physically drained most of the day
- energy starting to return late in the evening
- usually needing more than eight hours of sleep
- needing caffeine or other stimulants to function

- difficulties focusing, concentrating, and remembering
- reduced libido
- frequent colds and flu
- recovering from illnesses more slowly
- craving salty food
- mild anxiety and depression.

Adrenal fatigue sufferers may benefit from acupuncture, as it can improve adrenal function. The stress hormone cortisol is kept in a healthy range with treatments, while serotonin and dopamine production are also stimulated. Here's a testimony from a patient with adrenal fatigue: "I had too much stress in my life and didn't have enough energy to walk down the street. My adrenals were exhausted, and my liver and spleen were overloaded. Through a series of acupuncture treatments, I was able to heal in half the time it would normally take to recover. Acupuncture has helped me so much that not only can I walk down the street, but I'm in training to recertify as a fitness instructor. I could not have done this without acupuncture at a critical time in my health. I am extremely grateful, and I would recommend acupuncture to anyone."

Those with adrenal problems can also gain a lot from Chinese herbs. An herbal remedy created especially for you by your Chinese medicine practitioner is tailored to your symptoms and condition. Unlike caffeine or energy drinks, herbs won't give you a rapid, artificial energy boost or an adrenaline rush. This kind of fast release of adrenaline stimulation is frequently a contributing factor to adrenal exhaustion. Traditional Chinese medicines gradually strengthen your body from the inside out. Herbal tonic compositions will help your body repair what it has been losing over the years. They can reestablish wellness and natural energy by healing organ systems like the adrenals and kidneys. The combined practice reduces the negative effects of stress on the body and mind and strengthens the immune system as a whole.

Traditional Chinese medicine is among the more effective treatments for adrenal fatigue. With treatment, you can expect changes in mood, happiness, stress level, and digestion, as well as improved sleep and increased vitality. However, it will still be a while before any discernible changes in vigor are seen because adrenal exhaustion is a chronic condition that starts long before the symptoms begin to manifest. You can overcome adrenal exhaustion with persistence and patience.

Long-Haul COVID-19, Epstein-Barr Virus, and Chronic Fatigue Syndrome

Numerous medical diseases, such as long-haul COVID-19, Epstein-Barr virus, hypothyroidism, anemia, and depression, can cause fatigue as a symptom. Chronic Fatigue Syndrome (CFS), or myalgic encephalomyelitis (ME), may be indicated by persistent fatigue and intense exhaustion lasting longer than three to six months. This ailment makes it difficult to carry out daily tasks and function normally.

Although the exact causes of chronic fatigue are unknown, it is thought that chronic bacterial infections, severe candida overgrowth, viral infections such as long-haul COVID-19 and the Epstein-Barr virus (EBV, mono), immunological dysfunction, nutritional deficiencies, excessive stress, or a combination of these factors may be to blame.

There is so much going on in our lives today that it is understandable why many people feel overworked and tired all the time. Stress and sleep deprivation are so widespread that many people get weary easily. But when a person's level of exhaustion reaches the point where they never feel rested and find it difficult to carry out regular daily tasks, fatigue becomes a major health issue that needs to be addressed. Chronic fatigue is a mental and physical loss of energy that goes beyond simply feeling tired or experiencing normal sleepiness because it typically persists long after you rest. This total lack of energy can make even the simplest daily duties appear challenging. Physical or muscular weariness inhibits a person from using the body in the ways they are used to while being mentally weary results in sleepiness and the inability to focus the mind sufficiently to complete routine duties.

The medical world does not completely comprehend CFS as an illness; rather, it is recognized as a syndrome, which is a group of symptoms that are frequently observed together.

Some symptoms of CFS include:

- extreme tiredness that is exacerbated by physical or mental activity
- severe headaches
- heightened sensitivity to sounds, lights, and other constant stimuli
- cognitive dysfunction and brain fog
- feeling tired following a full night of sleep
- persistent throat pain
- tenderness in the lymph nodes
- persistent joint and muscle pain.

Chronic fatigue can be challenging for clinicians to diagnose with certainty, partly because the symptoms are "invisible" and subjective but also because there are other medical disorders with comparable symptoms, like fibromyalgia and lupus.

Because chronic fatigue is poorly understood, it can also be challenging to treat. There is currently no officially recognized specific allopathic medical treatment for chronic fatigue. Patients are generally told to take it easy, pace themselves while doing light activities, and learn to stay away from things that worsen their tiredness.

Doctors may prescribe antidepressants to treat mental instability and insomnia. However, these drugs can have adverse side effects and might lead to dependence. This emphasis on addressing CFS's symptoms rather than its underlying causes could result in extended misery.

If past therapies haven't brought you any relief, you are probably seeking other directions to take. Many chronic fatigue patients turn to acupuncture, and the results are compelling. "When I first began receiving acupuncture, I couldn't always walk. I was suffering from severe chronic fatigue to such an extent that my family thought I had MS, a disease that my grandmother had died of. I had seen 25 medical doctors to try to get help with my symptoms, and only one of them had helped me in a significant way. After I started acupuncture treatments, I began to see improvements in my symptoms. However, I was very resistant at first to some of the lifestyle changes recommended to me, particularly my diet, which I had thought was good enough. I have been anything BUT disappointed. I have dramatically improved. I no longer have severe weakness and tingling in my extremities; I no longer have terrible nerve symptoms like nausea, weird electrical pains, and TMJ; and I have resumed many activities that had been severely limited before by my fatigue. I know it's only up and up from here."

A study on the effects of acupuncture on chronic fatigue syndrome was conducted by researchers at the Beijing Chaoyang Fatou Community Health Service Center, comparing three groups. Patients in one group received sham acupuncture treatments (a placebo control system). Patients in the second group underwent standard acupuncture to treat chronic fatigue syndrome. The third group received both regular acupuncture and moxibustion therapy. The findings show that sham acupuncture does not significantly improve patient outcomes, but warm needling acupuncture and standard acupuncture do. (Lu et al., 2014).

Another paper in 2015 reported the results of a multicenter controlled trial in four hospitals on 150 participants with chronic fatigue syndrome or idiopathic chronic fatigue. Results showed that a 4-week course of acupuncture, in addition to usual care, could help improve fatigue in patients (Kim et al., 2023).

You can expect one to three treatments per week with acupuncture for fatigue. Acupuncture treats not just the symptoms of fatigue but the cause as well. Anyone can have a second cup of coffee or, even worse, down an energy drink every day. That strategy won't just fail to address your fatigue problems; over time, it will make them worse. On the other hand, methods like acupuncture, mindfulness, dietary adjustments, lifestyle changes, and qigong exercise—all recommended by your acupuncturist—may successfully end your chronic fatigue.

Allergies and Asthma

Asthma is a chronic disease characterized by chronic allergic airway inflammation. This illness causes symptoms in patients, such as coughing, wheezing, and breathing problems. Anti-inflammatory, anti-bronchial spasm, and anti-cough drugs, as well as oxygen, are used to manage this condition. Recent clinical investigations have shown that acupuncture can be used with traditional asthma treatment as a complementary therapy.

A recent systematic review evaluated nine studies on the effectiveness of conventional therapies combined with acupuncture for treating asthma in adults and adolescents. Results showed that the interleukin-6 (IL-6) blood levels, a potent indicator of disease activity, dropped drastically, and the symptom response rates improved (Jiang et al., 2019).

Acupuncture can also be helpful as a complementary treatment for other allergic diseases. A controlled multicenter trial on 422 people with hay fever showed that the use of antihistamines decreased and disease-specific quality of life significantly improved after acupuncture (Brinkhaus et al., 2013).

Autoimmune Disease: Crohn's Disease

Inflammation of the digestive tract can result in inflammatory bowel disease (IBD). This condition can take two rather similar forms: ulcerative colitis and Crohn's disease. Both forms can cause excruciating pain and discomfort and intestinal ulcers, but they can be controlled with medicine. Acupuncture is used as a complementary therapy in both forms of IBD. This means that the method only aids in the management of symptoms and does not treat the disease completely. Here, we take a look at acupuncture treatment for Crohn's disease.

Numerous studies back up the advantages of acupuncture for Crohn's disease. Some acupuncturists also use electroacupuncture in addition to traditional acupuncture. This technique entails applying a small electric current to the acupuncture needles, which activates a stronger response and stimulation. Moxibustion is sometimes used in conjunction with acupuncture to treat Crohn's disease. In this instance, the practitioner warms special sticks or burns herbs like mugwort over certain body areas.

A 2014 study on the effects of acupuncture and moxibustion on persons with Crohn's disease found that the symptoms had decreased after three weeks of treatments, three times per week. According to the study's findings, those who received acupuncture and moxibustion treatment had improved quality of life ratings and lower levels of Crohn's disease activity. 74% of patients receiving acupuncture and moxibustion had symptom remission after 12 weeks of treatment. In contrast, only 36% of the control group's patients were in remission, and no longer had symptoms (Bao, 2014).

According to a 2017 study, electroacupuncture treatment for Crohn's patients resulted in brain modifications that may have lessened their sense of pain and unpleasant feelings. For 12 weeks, participants received three electroacupuncture sessions per week and then underwent MRI scans to look for changes in the brain. The scientists discovered that electroacupuncture impacted a region of the brain that controls pain, particularly visceral pain, including stomach pain. The researchers came to the conclusion that electroacupuncture could assist in achieving brain-gut balance to lessen discomfort in those with Crohn's disease (Bao et al., 2017).

Irritable Bowel Syndrome (IBS)

IBS is a combination of abdominal pain or discomfort and issues with bowel movements, such as abnormal frequency or abnormally formed stools (hard, soft, or liquid). It could be a persistent issue that alters your way of living. People with IBS may skip work or school more frequently and feel less capable of engaging in regular activities. Some people may need to adjust their work environment by working from home, working fewer hours, or perhaps taking time off altogether. The illness affects around twice as many women as men. It is unclear why; however, some studies speculate that the fluctuating hormone levels during the menstrual cycle may be a factor. Bulking agents such as psyllium, antibiotics, and anti-spasm medicines are used to control IBS.

Acupuncture is widely used as a complementary therapy for IBS. According to studies, acupuncture may assist with stomach bloating as well as other IBS symptoms. A systematic review evaluated six clinical trials on the effects of acupuncture on IBS. The authors concluded that acupuncture significantly helped control IBS symptoms (Chao, 2014).

Nausea and Vomiting

Prevention of nausea and vomiting is one of the best-established applications of acupuncture. In fact, it was one of the first uses of acupuncture recognized by the NIH back in the nineties. It is thought that acupuncture exerts this effect by promoting the secretion of beta-endorphins and ACTH, which, in turn, block the vomiting center in the brain. There is a wealth of clinical studies confirming the efficacy of acupuncture in controlling nausea and vomiting induced by chemotherapy, morning sickness in pregnant women, and even motion sickness (Morehead & Salmon, 2020).

Motion sickness acupuncture treatments are offered on most cruise ships, and they are extremely successful, even when patches and motion sickness medications fail, as this patient experienced: "I had motion sickness despite having patches and taking Dramamine. The acupuncture worked the first time! I went back for two more sessions to stay feeling well. I would not hesitate to receive acupuncture again."

Morning sickness can be effectively treated and prevented with acupuncture. For some people, it might produce results relatively quickly. During the first trimester, it is preferable to have one or two acupuncture sessions every week, depending on how severe and frequent your morning sickness is and how quickly your body responds to the acupuncture treatment.

Nausea and vomiting are common anesthetic effects in the days and weeks following surgery. In a recent study, 97 hysterectomy patients were randomly assigned to two groups: an acupuncture group and a control group (no acupuncture). According to the study, acupuncture helped patients have less postoperative nausea (Pires et al., 2022).

In 2022, a paper in the *Phytomedicine* journal gave an overview of 51 systematic reviews on the effects of acupuncture on acupuncture for cancer-related complications. Each of these systematic reviews had distilled results from several studies. The authors concluded that acupuncture was beneficial to cancer survivors, improved their quality of life, and eased cancer-related issues, including nausea and vomiting in them (Zhang et al., 2022). As one of my patients said: "I have been getting acupuncture since late October, and I can't rave enough about it. I started chemo in mid-October, and it was miserable. Once I started receiving acupuncture twice a week, it really helped me recover quicker from each additional round of chemotherapy. I have continued to receive acupuncture, and it also helped considerably through my radiation."

Hypertension

The Yellow Emperor's classic on internal medicine said that consuming too much salt could result in a "hardened pulse" (He & Whelton, 2002). Acupuncture was used to treat this condition. The concept of hypertension has seen a long evolution since then. Chronic, severe hypertension can damage the brain, kidneys, and cardiovascular system. This is significant because most cases of hypertension are without symptoms and go undiagnosed until indications of organ damage appear. Modern medical treatment includes dietary and lifestyle modifications as well as medications like diuretics, calcium channel blockers, and ACE inhibitors.

Numerous studies show that, when used in conjunction with other therapies, acupuncture effectively lowers blood pressure (Sudhakaran, 2020). In such instances, the dosages of antihypertensive drugs can be gradually decreased, lowering their potential negative effects. In a trial involving 24 male and 10 female patients, researchers looked at the effects of acupuncture treatment on blood pressure in hypertension patients who had been receiving antihypertensive medication therapy for at least 24 months. Each patient was taking one to three antihypertensive drugs. After receiving acupuncture for one month every two days for a total of 15 sessions, the patients' systolic and diastolic blood pressures were significantly lowered. The authors recommended including acupuncture as a blood pressure-regulating method in the guidelines for treating hypertension (Çevik & İşeri, 2013).

Infertility

Several medical disorders that impact fertility can benefit from acupuncture. These include problems with the ovarian reserve and sperm quality, fibroids, endometriosis, and polycystic ovary syndrome (PCOS). It might also lessen some of the negative effects of fertility medication such as bloating and nausea.

Researchers examined data from numerous controlled studies in a systematic review of the efficacy of acupuncture on the polycystic ovarian syndrome. They discovered some evidence that acupuncture helps women with polycystic ovarian syndrome have better menstruation and ovulation. Researchers also found that using acupuncture in conjunction with prescription drugs led to small increases in hormone levels (Jo et al., 2017).

Menopause

Women experience a variety of symptoms during the transition to menopause, some of which may appear months or even years before they cease having regular monthly periods. The typical duration of menopause symptoms is four years; however, they can persist for up to 12 years. The most frequent of these signs are hot flushes, which can make you feel stressed, uncomfortable, and perspiring. Additionally, you can have mood swings, headaches, and sleep problems.

Acupuncture works by balancing hormones, which decreases the frequency and severity of these symptoms. It is a gentle and effective method of treating menopause symptoms. A recent clinical study showed that acupuncture could successfully treat menopausal symptoms. This is exciting because other medical treatments for menopausal symptoms are only modestly successful, and hormone treatment for those symptoms has fallen out of favor.

Researchers in the study monitored the outcomes for 70 menopausal women who either received weekly 15-minute acupuncture for five weeks or did not receive any. The study discovered that women who underwent acupuncture experienced much fewer hot flashes than those who did not. Additionally, patients who had acupuncture reported experiencing less intense and less frequent daytime and nighttime perspiration, generalized sweating, sleep issues, emotional and physical symptoms, and skin and hair issues. In total, 80% of the women who received acupuncture reported that the procedure had helped lessen their menopausal symptoms (Kamma Sundgaard Lund et al., 2019).

Menstrual Cramps and Premenstrual Syndrome

Premenstrual syndrome (PMS) afflicts many women of childbearing age in one way or another. It can present with physical, behavioral, and psychological symptoms. Symptoms can vary in severity. Physical symptoms can include headaches, nausea, breast tenderness and swelling, back pain, abdominal pain and bloating, muscle and joint pain, water retention, and weight gain. Emotional and behavioral symptoms may include irritability, anger, depressed mood, tearfulness, anxiety, fatigue, and insomnia.

Acupuncture treatments significantly lessen these symptoms as they help regulate hormones, calm the nerves, and relieve pain. Those whose lives are run by their cycles and PMS can reclaim their lives with acupuncture: "Initially, I came in for help with PMS symptoms, but I ended up feeling a big difference with my anxiety levels in addition to my PMS symptoms. After every session, I felt relaxed and ready to take on the world!"

In a 2018 study, 60 women between the ages of 17 and 23 were randomly assigned to either the study group or the control group. The study group had acupuncture for 20 minutes each day, 15 days per month, for a total of 90 days, while the control group did not get acupuncture. The results showed that acupuncture significantly reduced pain and menstrual cramps, headache, dizziness, diarrhea, fainting, mood swings, fatigue, nausea, and vomiting in those who received acupuncture treatment compared to those who did not (Shetty et al., 2018).

Sleep Disorders: Insomnia and Sleep Apnea

Although sleep is essential for overall health and normal daytime functioning, not everyone finds it easy to get enough sleep. Everyone occasionally has problems sleeping, but millions of American adults have trouble getting to sleep and staying asleep. You might be one of the 1 in 3 people who have insomnia. Lack of sleep makes it difficult for you to function during the day.

Adults should, on average, obtain 7–8 hours of sleep each night. When someone is sleep deprived for several days, they experience transient or acute weariness. However, studies reveal that more than a third of Americans usually sleep less than seven hours every night. In addition to leaving one feeling overly exhausted, poor sleeping patterns can result in various chronic health issues.

The signs of insomnia include difficulty falling asleep, difficulty getting back to sleep after waking up throughout the night, waking up early, and poor sleep quality. These symptoms can last from a few days to months or more. Insomnia has a variety of causes, including physical diseases like sleep apnea, mental health issues including anxiety and chronic pain, and irregular sleep schedules. However, in many instances, no specific physical, psychological, or environmental causes are found for insomnia.

The effects of insomnia on social harmony and emotional stability include fatigue, reduced function, cognitive decline, trouble in social interactions, tension, and worry. Long-term insomnia has been linked to depression and cardiovascular disease.

Sedative medications are the mainstay of insomnia treatment. These may occasionally provide short-term advantages, but continued usage can have negative effects such as lethargy, addiction, and neurological harm.

Acupuncture has long been utilized in Traditional Chinese Medicine to improve sleeplessness. It was understood to be accomplished through restoring normal function and achieving mental and physical balance. In modern times, it is becoming more widely recognized as a helpful complementary treatment for insomnia. It has been demonstrated in numerous clinical trials to be a successful treatment for sleeplessness.

Compared to sleep medications, acupuncture is often more accessible and has fewer adverse effects. Some sedatives that are frequently used to treat insomnia can make a person feel sleepy the next day, impair their cognitive function, or make them dependent on the drug. The potential benefits of acupuncture for sleeping disorders make it an excellent complementary treatment, and it can also be used safely in conjunction with other sleep treatments.

Sleep problems are more common among people with anxiety and depression. Acupuncture has proven to be effective in treating insomnia in special situations, for example, in people with depression and those suffering from chronic pain.

A 2019 evaluation of nine studies including almost 1,000 patients with chronic pain-related insomnia found that acupuncture was more effective at enhancing sleep quality than a placebo or medication (Liu et al., 2019).

Improvement in sleep quality leads to better overall health. It is one of the hallmarks of receiving regular acupuncture treatments: "I'm enjoying my acupuncture session and have been getting great results. Overall, I feel more balanced physically and emotionally, with additional improvements in my sleep quality and a decrease in muscle pain. The sessions are very peaceful. I really look forward to them!"

Acupuncture may also be effective for some suffering from Sleep Apnea. In obstructive sleep apnea, the patient temporarily stops breathing while sleeping. It can lead to oxygen deprivation throughout the night, making one tired the next day. According to an analysis of nine studies involving nearly 600 patients, the symptoms of sleep apnea, drowsiness, and oxygen saturation levels were all significantly improved by acupuncture, particularly among those with moderate to severe cases (Wang et al., 2023).

According to the research, acupuncture may help treat insomnia through several pathways. These include:

- increasing melatonin production, the hormone that controls the sleep cycle

- controlling the amounts of neurotransmitters such as dopamine, serotonin, GABA, and neuropeptide Y helps to relax and de-stress the body and mind

- increasing nitric oxide helps the brain operate normally, promotes mental relaxation, and enhances sleep
- reducing the fight-or-flight response and sympathetic nervous system activity increases body calmness and relaxation
- increasing blood flow helps the body and mind unwind and enhance sleep.

Addiction

Each person with addiction has unique requirements and circumstances. Therefore, treatments that are effective for one individual may not be effective for another. This is why it is advised to combine complementary therapies with counseling and a full detox.

Since its introduction as a way of treating addiction in the 1970s at the Lincoln Memorial Hospital in New York, acupuncture has been used to treat addiction to a variety of substances. The medical staff at this hospital found acupuncture to be so successful in treating heroin addiction that they stopped providing methadone and started using acupuncture instead. As a result, one of the doctors at Lincoln Memorial Hospital, Michael O. Smith, founded the National Acupuncture Detoxification Association (NADA) in 1985.

Acupuncture is increasingly used as a supplemental therapy in numerous addiction rehabilitation programs. Substance addiction cannot be treated solely with acupuncture. It is utilized in conjunction with other recovery techniques like psychotherapy, 12-step programs, group counseling, or complementary and alternative therapies like yoga, meditation, and art therapy.

The first step in using acupuncture for addiction is always to find out if you have any underlying medical issues that might be causing you pain and driving you to self-medicate with tobacco, alcohol, or drugs. If that is the case, acupuncture can be used to address those specific health issues and relieve pain there as well.

The World Health Organization has accepted the use of acupuncture in treating addiction, and there is research to support the effectiveness of acupuncture in treating addiction. For instance, a study on 40 addicts found that acupuncture reduced the withdrawal symptoms linked to Rapid Opiate Detoxification (Montazeri et al., 2002). Acupuncture has the advantages of being affordable, safe, and having no side effects.

Some of the advantages of acupuncture for the supportive treatment of addiction are the following:

- fewer cravings
- a decrease in withdrawal signs
- reduced dependence on prescription drugs
- lower levels of anxiety
- a better sense of serenity
- lower stress levels
- heightened relaxation
- an enhanced feeling of well-being
- a renewed sense of energy
- better sleeping habits
- an increase in cooperative attitudes
- higher levels of control
- diminished rage and mood swings
- fewer severe panic attacks.

The minor possibility that acupuncture may not be effective for all people with addiction appears insignificant when one considers that all of these benefits can be gained without using drugs or prescription medication.

The exact mechanism of acupuncture's action in addiction is unknown. Drugs and other addictive substances influence the dopaminergic system in the brain and cause sensations of pleasure and euphoria, which promote continuous use. Drugs also reinforce continuing use by suppressing withdrawal symptoms like dysphoria. These effects of addictive substances are thought to be lessened by acupuncture, thus reducing drug use (Lin et al., 2012).

Acupuncture treatment is thought to lessen the positive reinforcing effects of drugs by reducing the quantity of dopamine released when a drug is used. The "high" or "buzz" is lessened without the dopamine spike, and the person is less likely to use the substance again. On the other hand, acupuncture inhibits GABA neurons, which causes an increase in dopamine production. The influx of dopamine into specific brain regions elevates mood and lessens withdrawal symptoms, such as dysphoria and distress. Otherwise, a user would try taking more of the addictive substance to ease withdrawal.

Stress

In today's world, there's very little we can do to avoid stress completely. It affects everyone. We all experience stress, whether it comes from an external stressor like work, family, friends, or relationships; a bodily stressor like inactivity, overactivity, a poor diet, or disease symptoms; or a psychological stressor like anxiety or despair. It may reach a level that can lead to physical or psychological disorders.

In a broader context, stress is a normal aspect of human life. We are able to respond to emergencies and provide results swiftly in a moment of high demand thanks to our innate stress responses, which include elevated heart rate and blood pressure, improved mental clarity, and heightened focus. In modest doses, stress can make us feel alive and engaged and lead to successful results. However, if stress is a continuous companion, the stress chemicals our systems release (cortisol, adrenaline, and norepinephrine) can be harmful over time.

Chronic stress may have the following common effects:

- constant worries, agitation, and racing thoughts
- forgetfulness, trouble focusing, and difficulty making decisions
- difficulty sleeping
- lethargy
- diminished sexual function or a loss of libido
- migraines and headaches
- clenched jaw or teeth grinding
- sore, strained muscles, especially in the neck and shoulders
- changes in appetite
- nausea, diarrhea, constipation, heartburn, or other digestive discomforts
- rapid heartbeat.

Chronic stress raises your chances for depression, anxiety, and more severe gut issues like colitis, inflammatory bowel disease, gastroesophageal reflux disease, heart attacks, heart disease, eating disorders, and obesity.

Conventional therapies for stress include prescription pharmaceuticals such as anti-anxiety medications, as well as, to a much lesser extent, cognitive behavioral therapy, and relaxation techniques. Some people may benefit from anti-anxiety drugs, but they can have side effects that are stressful in and of themselves. Cognitive behavioral therapy can be helpful for some psychological issues and aid in relaxation in some cases. However, it is not very effective for the physiological effects of stress, which, if not also treated, can increase stress or lessen the effectiveness of the therapy. Relaxation techniques can be beneficial but may be difficult at first or take considerable time to take effect.

Unlike drugs, acupuncture has been shown to be safe and does not carry any risks. Few studies have examined the direct effects of acupuncture on stress, but there is much evidence demonstrating the treatment's benefits for illnesses related to stress, such as sleeplessness, anxiety and depression, headaches and migraines, post-traumatic stress disorder, and even stress-related incontinence. The World Health Organization recommends acupuncture for several of these illnesses.

Acupuncture can reduce stress through several processes, according to research. It works on parts of the brain that are known to lessen sensitivity to pain and stress. It also encourages relaxation and turns off the "analytical" brain, which is involved in worry and anxiety.

Stress activates the sympathetic nervous system, whereas acupuncture can activate the opposing parasympathetic nervous system, which starts the relaxation response. Acupuncture alters the brain's chemistry to assist in fighting depressive moods by lowering serum levels of cortisol and regulating levels of neurotransmitters and hormones such as serotonin, dopamine, GABA, and ACTH. Acupuncture decreases inflammation by encouraging the release of vascular and immunomodulatory substances and restoring pathological alterations in inflammatory cytokine levels linked to stress responses.

Anger and Irritability

Frequent anger-related emotions can have a variety of negative effects on the body. Blood pressure, body temperature, and heart rate all rise when one is angry. Myocardial ischemia, a lack of oxygen in the heart's pumping muscles, is also more likely to occur. This can result in heart attacks, blocked arteries, and other cardiovascular disease-related health issues.

In some people, anger can become more than a passing emotion and develop into a personality trait. For these people, anger becomes the default emotion when responding to emotionally charged events or fears. In these instances, anger can negatively impact relationships, daily life, and mental health because it frequently includes other negative emotions like hostility and aggression.

According to Traditional Chinese Medicine, patterns of disharmony involving the liver are connected to anger and irritability. Removing energy blockages can help prevent the development of emotional issues like anger.

Consider acupuncture for anger and irritability. Traditional Chinese Medicine, including acupuncture, can help people who are stressed, angry, or frustrated. Regular acupuncture sessions help resolve minor irritations before they develop into more serious issues.

Acupuncture strives to restore balance to your body, mind, and spirit through a series of customized sessions. The neuro-endocrine-immune network, which controls the body's regulatory system, and the pathways that control the acute stress response are modulated by acupuncture. While there is little scientific information on how acupuncture particularly treats anger in the body, it has shown promise in treating it along with other emotional disorders like PTSD, anxiety, and depression. By discussing your objectives with your acupuncturist, you will be able to develop a tailored treatment plan to address your concerns regarding anger and irritability.

Traditional Chinese Medicine offers many lifestyle and dietary recommendations for managing anger:

- **Avoid recreational drug use**: Excessive alcohol use might impair your ability to cope with frustration.

- **Increase your outdoor activity levels**: If you are feeling agitated, spend time in nature. Go trekking or learn to play golf.

- **Stretch**: Make time for a morning stretch in your schedule. Traditional Chinese Medicine believes that the liver stores blood during times of rest and releases it during times of activity.

- **Eat greens**: Young plants, such as sprouts and fresh herbs, as well as fresh, leafy greens, can help the liver perform better.

- **Try something sour**: Add lemon slices to your water, top your salad with vinegar and olive oil, and add a piece of dill pickle to your meal.

- **Enjoy milk thistle tea**: Milk thistle tea enhances the liver's ability to rid the body of harmful chemicals such as alcohol, drugs, pesticides, environmental pollutants, and even heavy metals like mercury. It also helps protect liver cells from these toxins.

Anxiety

Anxiety is an emotional reaction to stress that causes you to feel scared, anxious, or hesitant about things like beginning a new job or speaking in public. Most people will occasionally feel anxious during difficult times at some point in their lives; nevertheless, persistent anxiety is abnormal and has to be managed. Psychotherapy, medicines, or a mix of the two are frequently used to treat it.

In the U.S., anxiety problems affect over 40 million adults (National Alliance on Mental Illness, 2017). People suffering from anxiety frequently experience feelings of dread or fear, as well as irrational or racing thoughts. In order to avoid an anxiety episode, people who suffer from anxiety often avoid particular situations or people. In addition to mental changes, anxiety can cause shaking, muscle tightness, shallow breathing, an elevated heart rate, and sweating.

Anxiety disorders are characterized by overwhelming worry and fear about commonplace events, come in different forms, and may have a sudden onset, as experienced by this patient: "I've had a fear of falling for the last year. I've only been able to navigate by being able to touch a wall or object. Being outdoors and attempting to walk was paralyzing. I managed by clutching my husband's arm or carrying a cane. Five sessions of acupuncture seem to have removed my irrational fear. I suffered from post-traumatic stress disorder (PTSD), and acupuncture seems to have removed this demon from my mind. I highly recommend that anyone give it a try."

Various forms of anxiety disorders include:

- **Post-traumatic stress disorder (PTSD)** is a form of anxiety that appears after a traumatic experience, such as a physical or sexual attack, an accident, or a traumatic incident during military service.

- **Generalized anxiety disorder (GAD)** is a chronic anxiety condition in which you experience fear or worry most of the time; this feeling is frequently unprovoked and occurs for no discernible reason.

- **Panic attacks** are intense anxiety episodes that can develop suddenly and cause extreme fear and physical symptoms, including a racing heart, dizziness, dry mouth, trembling, and nausea.

- **Social phobia** is overwhelming anxiety and self-consciousness brought on by social events such as public speaking, eating, or drinking in front of others, or meeting new people.

- **Obsessive-compulsive disorder (OCD)** is marked by compulsive habits like counting, hand washing, and cleaning.

Although the precise cause of anxiety disorder is uncertain, traumatic events and life experiences are thought to be the main triggers. It is believed that some people are more prone to anxiety due to inherited features (carrying particular genes) and certain personalities (such as perfectionists or timid/shy personalities). Anxiety can also be brought on by some medications, poor health, and medical illnesses like diabetes, an overactive thyroid, heart disease, lung ailments (asthma, COPD), and chronic pain.

The following life experiences are among the triggers for anxiety disorders:

- persistent stress
- harassment or social exclusion
- being in a toxic relationship
- experiencing a relationship breakup
- passing away of a family member
- worries about money or your job
- childhood or adult abuse, or trauma
- alcohol, recreational drugs, and energy drinks.

Acupuncturists successfully treat anxiety using acupuncture, herbology, lifestyle recommendations, and even nutrition. Frequent treatments help reduce stress and promote relaxation. The impact of acupuncture on anxiety has been the subject of numerous investigations. According to these studies, which mainly focus on generalized anxiety disorder, acupuncture may be effective in treating anxiety.

For instance, a 2015 study discovered that acupuncture reduced symptoms in individuals with anxiety who did not react to other therapies, such as psychotherapy and medication. For 10 weeks, participants received 10 acupuncture sessions of 30 minutes each. Even 10 weeks after the end of the treatment, they reported a considerable decrease in their anxiety (Errington-Evans, 2023). In a 2016 study, anxiety related hormones were found to be reduced by acupuncture in rats. According to the researchers, acupuncture may affect how the animal body initiates the fight-or-flight response (Yao et al., 2016).

A comprehensive review and meta-analysis of randomized controlled trials published in English and Chinese were conducted in 2021 to determine if acupuncture benefits anxiety disorders. This review includes 20 clinical trials, 18 of which were published in Chinese, and all included individuals with generalized anxiety disorder. Acupuncture was found to be helpful in managing anxiety symptoms. It also demonstrated good tolerability and safety in the treatment of anxiety disorders. The data is promising for acupuncture as a practical and secure choice, even though we still need to learn more about how exactly it impacts anxiety disorder (Yang et al., 2021).

Acupuncture activates the natural relaxation response and the parasympathetic nervous system explaining the possible physiological mechanisms by which the positive effects of acupuncture in relieving anxiety are brought about. Acupuncture activates the natural relaxation response and the parasympathetic nervous system. Our sympathetic nervous system activates in response to stress, causing a range of physiological and emotional changes in the body, including anxiety. The parasympathetic nervous system works as a brake, slowing down the nervous system and promoting relaxation.

Anxiety and emotional problems can make the immune system less effective and cause more inflammation in the body. Acupuncture has been demonstrated to restore immunological function when anxiety is present by controlling the release of inflammatory chemicals. Cortisol and adrenaline are two hormones that are produced in response to stress to help the body respond to it appropriately. Serotonin, the hormone linked to happiness and a sense of wellness, can be depleted by prolonged stress. Acupuncture can balance these hormones and lessen anxiety symptoms by harmonizing neurotransmitters and hormones that ease stress.

Finally, acupuncture may reduce stress and pain sensitivity by acting on the brain's somatosensory cortex. It may also make the "analytical" brain cortex, which is responsible for worrying thoughts, less active.

Depression

Depression, sometimes known as "major depressive disorder," is a condition marked by a persistent sense of melancholy and a loss of interest or pleasure. There could be a few more symptoms as well:

- alterations in appetite and weight
- fatigue and insufficient energy
- difficulty concentrating, making decisions, and remembering things
- difficulty falling asleep or excessive sleep
- frustration and irritability, especially over trivial issues
- guilt or a sense of worthlessness
- suicidal or death-related ideas.

Medication, psychotherapy (talk therapy), or a combination of the two are frequently used to treat depression, with varying results. Despite continued treatment, many patients will continue to experience depression and are interested in alternative treatments like acupuncture. One reason is that acupuncture, unlike antidepressants, has almost no adverse effects. Research supports the usefulness of acupuncture as a treatment for depression and its associated symptoms. Herbology is also very successful in addressing treatments. Unlike antidepressants, Traditional Chinese herbal formulas do not suppress your emotions but strengthen you to support your coping mechanisms.

Numerous studies have indicated that acupuncture may be effective in managing depression symptoms. For instance, in an 8-week acupuncture trial involving 151 men and women, researchers discovered that depressive symptoms considerably improved. Irrespective of whether the acupuncture was targeted or general, individuals who received it fared better than those who did not (Manber et al., 2023).

An extensive review examined 64 acupuncture for depression studies involving more than 7,100 participants, and it was published in the Cochrane Database of Systematic Reviews. It was discovered that acupuncture was helpful in lowering the severity of depression compared to other depression treatments or no treatment at all (Smith et al., 2018).

A significant percentage of pregnant women may experience depression. The mother's depression may harm both the mother and the fetus during pregnancy. Antidepressants may cause some pregnant women to worry and turn to alternative therapies instead, and pregnancy-related depression responds well to acupuncture.

In a study, depressed pregnant women got acupuncture treatment specifically for depression for eight weeks, while another group received general acupuncture. Prenatal massages were given to a third group of pregnant women. The women who received the depression-specific acupuncture experienced a higher reduction in depressive symptoms compared to those who received the other treatments (Manber et al., 2023).

It is best to try acupuncture in conjunction with talk therapy, medicine, or other therapeutic modalities. The advantages of therapy, medication, or other medical care may be enhanced when used in conjunction with acupuncture as a complementary treatment. A systematic review of 29 studies on approximately 2,300 individuals, published in the Journal of Clinical Medicine, revealed that acupuncture was an effective supplement to conventional depression treatments (Armour et al., 2019).

Research suggests that acupuncture may be helpful when taken with antidepressant drugs. According to a literature review, antidepressants and acupuncture may work better together than antidepressants alone to treat depression (Chan et al., 2015).

Lack of energy is a typical sign of depression, and boosting the flow of qi, or vital energy is one of acupuncture's main goals in order to restore equilibrium in the body. Acupuncture is also frequently used to treat pain, which can either be the cause of depression or contribute to it.

Disturbances in the neuroendocrine system and the hypothalamic-pituitary-adrenal axis are related to the pathophysiology of depression. Acupuncture may improve depressive symptoms by controlling these disturbances. In mood disorders like depression, important brain, and central nervous system substances become imbalanced. Endogenous opioids and opioid receptors are some of these substances. Acupuncture may potentially help treat depression by regulating these components. Acupuncture raises dopamine and serotonin levels in the brain. An increase in these compounds can provide the body and mind with a boost, which might reduce certain symptoms of depression.

Grief

Grief is a normal response to a significant loss or bereavement. Less acute emotions like longing or regret sometimes accompany the loss of important belongings or missed opportunities and goals. Physical symptoms like headaches, tiredness, digestive issues, sinus or chest infections, and exhaustion can all result from grief.

We all encounter loss, change, and grief at some point in our lives. The loss of a close relative or other loved one is the most well-known cause of grief, as there is no doubt that such a loss causes tremendous sorrow and suffering. We are all familiar with this kind of loss, but there are other types of grief, too.

Consider the moment when you finally accomplish a goal you have been striving for, and BOOM! You succeed. You are at the mountain's peak. Have you ever achieved that kind of goal-oriented success? If so, have you observed that relatively quickly, after the rush and adrenaline of the triumph wear off, you start to wonder, "Now what?" You can experience disappointment when there is no longer a goal to serve as a motivating factor. In effect, it is a type of loss that can sometimes lead to grief.

The COVID-19 pandemic brought on unusual forms of grief. Many people were affected by the deaths of loved ones, yet they couldn't express grief in normal ways. Healthcare workers and their families experienced severe mental and physical stress due to the lack of support. These events have produced a distinctive form of grief. One that makes it more difficult to come to terms with the loss due to a general sense of unjustified absence, posttraumatic stress disorder, or survivor's guilt. As a result, the grieving process may spiral out of control.

Each of us processes loss differently and has distinct stages of reaction. At the same time, there are typically five recognizable stages of grief: denial, anger, bargaining, depression, and acceptance. Even though these feelings can coexist, one of them usually stands out more than the others, and the stages can cycle or reoccur. Sometimes we merely go through the motions, not even realizing the stages are happening.

Traditional Chinese Medicine offers the best foundation for treating patients who are experiencing this kind of pain because it sees the mind, body, and spirit as a single interconnected system. Acupuncture considers each emotion to be connected to specific regions of the body. Grief is particularly correlated with the respiratory system and lungs. The acupuncturist concentrates especially on the lung meridians or imbalances of the lungs while treating grief.

Acupuncture boosts and moves qi. Qi is consumed in times of grief, producing a void or a sense of emptiness and hollowness. Extreme emotion can also obstruct the free passage of qi; for instance, mourning is frequently felt in the chest, where the blocked qi causes one to feel as though they are "choking up." Acupuncture can help you recuperate in mind, body, and spirit under these situations by strengthening you and restoring balance and circulation to help you cope more easily.

Acupuncture is a safe alternative to antidepressants. Individuals trying to cope with the grieving process can try acupuncture without being concerned about any negative effects or adding this anxiety to their existing worries.

You can combine acupuncture with going to a talk therapist, practicing mindfulness meditation, or doing any number of other things in order to help you deal with grief. It's best to visit the acupuncturist soon after a bereavement or relationship split when you need assistance managing the overwhelming emotions of sadness and grief. Acupuncture cannot quickly remove feelings of grief and despair, but it can help with the healing process and encourage you to let go rather than become stuck.

Brain Fog

Brain power and clarity can give you significant advantages in life by enhancing your productivity, willpower, sense of connection to others, and ability to concentrate on your objectives. During periods of high stress and continual distraction, it is easy to feel as though our brains are having trouble keeping up with the demands of daily living, but if this condition becomes chronic, it may develop into "brain fog" or "mental fog."

Brain fog is a common condition brought on by various medical disorders. COVID-19, EBV, other persistent viruses, bacterial diseases like Lyme disease, autoimmune disorders such as Hashimoto's disease, anxiety, depression, chronic fatigue syndrome, menopause, and perimenopause are just a few of these conditions. Acupuncture lessens brain fog by addressing the underlying cause of the disease in addition to nourishing the brain, boosting blood flow to the head, and reducing emotional stress.

Brain fog symptoms include difficulty processing information, poor memory, difficulty focusing, and disorganized thought patterns. Simply put, "brain fog" is the inability to think clearly. You can feel disoriented, struggle to concentrate on a particular task, or feel mentally disorganized with your thoughts racing all over the place. Brain fog can also result in the inability to recall details like someone's name, what you had for lunch the day before, or where you put your keys.

An activity that used to be completed in 10 minutes with little effort may now take more than half an hour of focused effort. Frustration and fear are common responses to this situation. You may ask yourself, "How will I manage my life if I can't think?"

Many COVID-19 patients report persistent brain fog symptoms. The majority of people with autoimmune illnesses also have trouble focusing. They frequently struggle to concentrate on even the most straightforward jobs, assemble their thoughts, and complete the task at hand precisely. As a result, individuals often experience confusion and make errors.

Your ability to converse and write can both be impacted by brain fog. For instance, it can be challenging to choose the appropriate word to employ in a phrase when suffering from brain fog. You are aware of the word but cannot remember it. In certain circumstances, brain fog even causes short-term memory loss.

In a brain fog, managing numerous things at once is difficult due to poor focus and laborious thought. You may feel overwhelmed while executing simple activities and notice a decline in efficiency and performance levels due to your brain's difficulty focusing on multiple things simultaneously.

To deal with brain fog, you should first go through a complete medical workup for any underlying medical causes. In addition, there are several things you may do to sharpen your mind and recover mental clarity. You can accomplish this in a gentle and effective way by regularly having acupuncture. Studies conducted to determine the effect of acupuncture on brain fog symptoms have shown that acupuncture can relieve these symptoms.

Acupuncture practitioners can assist you in improving your capacity for clear thought. Many factors can contribute to brain fog, and acupuncturists often follow a multi-pronged approach to the treatment. In cases of brain fog, acupuncture places particular emphasis on re-establishing the balance of the body and mind and strengthening the spleen. When this balance is present, the mind and body communicate effectively to produce clear thoughts and efficient activities. We perform at our best and feel stronger, happier, and more confident at such times. Acupuncture also helps to lessen brain fog by treating the underlying disease causing the issue; for instance, a person who is suffering from extreme anxiety may also have incapacitating brain fog.

Weight Management

There is not much scientific evidence that using acupuncture alone will cause weight loss. The value of acupuncture, however, is potentially quite significant because studies suggest that acupuncture may aid in boosting metabolism, reducing appetite, and lowering stress hormone levels, all of which have an impact on calorie burn, snacking, and food preferences.

Many people who have trouble keeping their weight in check report being stress eaters. Overeating and eventual weight gain are intimately correlated with anxiety and stress. Stress hormones, including cortisol and adrenaline, are released by the body when it is under stress. Both hormones are crucial for survival in a fight-or-flight scenario. However, the body regularly releases these hormones in today's world of crammed schedules, work deadlines, and ever-changing newsreels, leading to several health disorders. As a result of the persistent stress reaction and hormone release, the body constantly craves carbs and sugars, overeats, and puts on weight.

Since acupuncture is very effective at controlling stress, it helps your body blunt the stress-related sympathetic response and activates the opposing parasympathetic, which is associated with relaxation. Furthermore, acupuncture promotes the release of endorphins, your "feel-good" hormones that support mood regulation. Many individuals use acupuncture to treat stress, anxiety, and depression. This is one of the key reasons acupuncture is thought to benefit people who are having trouble losing weight and managing their obesity.

Acupuncture, like any complementary therapy used for weight loss, will work best when joined by lifestyle changes, particularly a balanced diet, and exercise. In fact, a recent study indicated that acupuncture could help people lose weight significantly when combined with a 2,000-calorie diet and a 15-minute daily walk. In this 6-week research, those who had weekly acupuncture dropped an average of 10 lbs, compared to 3 lbs for those who didn't (Abdi et al., 2023).

Acupuncture's influence on your weight loss objectives extends beyond addressing weight. You might unintentionally eat more balanced meals, sleep better, or feel more relaxed as a result of receiving acupuncture. A patient struggling with a constant abundance of delicious temptations on the cruise ship wrote: "Because I have battled a lifelong weight problem, I decided to try acupuncture. Not knowing that my chemotherapy eleven years ago was also contributing to my many issues: dry mouth, mouth sores, sleeplessness, and knee pain. After three treatments with acupuncture these past two weeks, I am feeling much better and am not constantly hungry, even with the wonderful offerings on this cruise!"

Conclusion

Have you found yourself resonating with parts of this book? Have you been brushing aside nagging health concerns? Do you feel just OK and blame it on age, genetics, an old injury, or your environment? Wouldn't you want to feel better than just *okay*, feel your best, or maybe even Super Bowl fit?

Perhaps now, more than ever, is the time to shift our focus from treating disease to promoting wellness—doing so is both more effective and more economical than waiting for a disease to develop and become symptomatic. Health and vitality are not just the absence of symptoms. Traditional Chinese Medicine sets the bar higher. It understands that being well involves feeling physically energetic, mentally alert, emotionally balanced, capable of enjoying the quality of life that you desire, taking control of your health, and proactively maintaining it at its optimal peak.

I have written this book because I could not get a commercial spot on the Super Bowl or your local major sporting event. It is my way of promoting what has been life-changing for me and many others who have embraced a time-tested ancient medicine that is as relevant today as it was thousands of years ago. Acupuncture is powerful because it restores balance and harnesses your own body's healing ability safely and naturally.

I hope this book has piqued your interest enough to give acupuncture a try—it may well transform your life!

References

Abdi, H., Zhao, B., Darbandi, M., Ghayour-Mobarhan, M., Tavallaie, S., Rahsepar, A. A., Parizadeh, S. M. R., Safariyan, M., Nemati, M., Mohammadi, M., Abbasi-Parizad, P., Darbandi, S., Akhlaghi, S., & Ferns, G. A. A. (2023). The effects of body acupuncture on obesity: Anthropometric parameters, lipid profile, and inflammatory and immunologic markers. *The Scientific World Journal*, 2012, 1–11. https://doi.org/10.1100/2012/603539

Acupuncture Evidence Project. (2017). *The acupuncture evidence project*. Acupuncture.org.au. https://www.acupuncture.org.au/resources/publications/the-acupuncture-evidence-project

Armour, M., Ee, C. C., Hao, J., Wilson, T. M., Yao, S. S., & Smith, C. A. (2018). Acupuncture and acupressure for premenstrual syndrome. *Cochrane Database of Systematic Reviews*, 8. https://doi.org/10.1002/14651858.cd005290.pub2

Armour, M., Smith, C. A., Wang, L.-Q., Naidoo, D., Yang, G.-Y., MacPherson, H., Lee, M. S., & Hay, P. (2019). Acupuncture for depression: A systematic review and meta-analysis. *Journal of Clinical Medicine*, *8*(8), 1140. https://doi.org/10.3390/jcm8081140

Acupuncture: Review and analysis of reports on controlled clinical trials. (2003). World Health Organization. https://chiro.org/acupuncture/FULL/Acupuncture_WHO_2003.pdf

Bao, C., Wang, D., Liu, P., Shi, Y., Jin, X., Wu, L., Zeng, X., Zhang, J., Liu, H., & Wu, H. (2017). Effect of electro-acupuncture and moxibustion on brain connectivity in patients with Crohn's disease: A resting-state fMRI study. *Frontiers in Human Neuroscience*, 11. https://doi.org/10.3389/fnhum.2017.00559

Bao, C.-H. (2014). Randomized controlled trial: Moxibustion and acupuncture for the treatment of Crohn's disease. *World Journal of Gastroenterology*, *20*(31), 11000. https://doi.org/10.3748/wjg.v20.i31.11000

Brinkhaus, B., Ortiz, M., Witt, C. M., Roll, S., Linde, K., Pfab, F., Niggemann, B., Hummelsberger, J., Treszl, A., Ring, J., Zuberbier, T., Wegscheider, K., & Willich, S. N. (2013). Acupuncture in patients with seasonal allergic rhinitis. *Annals of Internal Medicine*, *158*(4), 225. https://doi.org/10.7326/0003-4819-158-4-201302190-00002

Cao, H., Pan, X., Li, H., & Liu, J. (2009). Acupuncture for treatment of insomnia: A Systematic Review of Randomized Controlled Trials. *The Journal of Alternative and Complementary Medicine*, *15*(11), 1171–1186. https://doi.org/10.1089/acm.2009.0041

Çevik, C., & İşeri, S. Ö. (2013). The effect of acupuncture on high blood pressure of patients using antihypertensive drugs. *Acupuncture & Electro-Therapeutics Research*, *38*(1), 1–15. https://doi.org/10.3727/036012913x13831831849448

Chan, Y.-Y., Lo, W.-Y., Yang, S.-N., Chen, Y.-H., & Lin, J.-G. (2015). The benefit of combined acupuncture and antidepressant medication for depression: A systematic review and meta-analysis. *Journal of Affective Disorders*, 176, 106–117. https://doi.org/10.1016/j.jad.2015.01.048

Chao, G.-Q. (2014). Effectiveness of acupuncture to treat irritable bowel syndrome: A meta-analysis. *World Journal of Gastroenterology*, *20*(7), 1871. https://doi.org/10.3748/wjg.v20.i7.1871

Chou, P.-C., & Chu, H.-Y. (2018). Clinical efficacy of acupuncture on rheumatoid arthritis and associated mechanisms: A systemic review. *Evidence-Based Complementary and Alternative Medicine*, 2018, 1–21. https://doi.org/10.1155/2018/8596918

Constitution of the world health organization. (1946). World Health Organization. https://www.who.int/about/governance/constitution

Department of Consumer Affairs Acupuncture Board. (2023). *License requirements - California acupuncture board.* Acupuncture.ca.gov. https://www.acupuncture.ca.gov/students/lic_require.shtml

Dias Junior, J. C. (2019). *Acupuncture in prevention, treatment of injuries and improvement of performance in athletes: Literature review.* Revista Científica Multidisciplinar Núcleo Do Conhecimento. https://www.nucleodoconhecimento.com.br/health/acupuncture-in-prevention

Dimitrova, A. (2017). Introducing a standardized acupuncture protocol for peripheral neuropathy: A case series. *Medical Acupuncture, 29*(6), 352–365. https://doi.org/10.1089/acu.2017.1242

Errington-Evans, N. (2023). Randomised controlled trial on the use of acupuncture in adults with chronic, non-responding anxiety symptoms. *Acupuncture in Medicine, 33*(2), 98–102. https://doi.org/10.1136/acupmed-2014-010524

Fani Marvasti, F., & Stafford, R. S. (2012). From sick care to health care — Reengineering prevention into the U.S. system. *New England Journal of Medicine, 367*(10), 889–891. https://doi.org/10.1056/nejmp1206230

Ghose, T. (2018). *Ötzi the Iceman's tattoos may have been a primitive form of acupuncture.* Livescience.com. https://www.livescience.com/63682-otzi-ice-man-took-medical-treatment.html

He, J., & Whelton, P. K. (2002). Commentary: Salt intake, hypertension and risk of cardiovascular disease: An important public health challenge. *International Journal of Epidemiology, 31*(2), 327–331. https://doi.org/10.1093/ije/31.2.327

Hochberg, M. C., Altman, R. D., April, K. T., Benkhalti, M., Guyatt, G., McGowan, J., Towheed, T., Welch, V., Wells, G., &

Tugwell, P. (2012). American college of rheumatology 2012 recommendations for the use of nonpharmacologic and pharmacologic therapies in osteoarthritis of the hand, hip, and knee. *Arthritis Care & Research*, *64*(4), 465–474. https://doi.org/10.1002/acr.21596

Jiang, C., Jiang, L., & Qin, Q. (2019). Conventional treatments plus acupuncture for asthma in adults and adolescent: A systematic review and meta-analysis. *Evidence-Based Complementary and Alternative Medicine*, 2019, 1–10. https://doi.org/10.1155/2019/9580670

Jo, J., Lee, Y. J., & Lee, H. (2017). Acupuncture for polycystic ovarian syndrome. *Medicine*, *96*(23), e7066. https://doi.org/10.1097/md.0000000000007066

Kamma Sundgaard Lund, Volkert Siersma, Brodersen, J., & Frans Boch Waldorff. (2019). Efficacy of a standardised acupuncture approach for women with bothersome menopausal symptoms: A pragmatic randomised study in primary care (the ACOM study). *BMJ Open*, *9*(1), e023637. https://doi.org/10.1136/bmjopen-2018-023637

Kim, J.-E., Seo, B.-K., Choi, J.-B., Kim, H.-J., Kim, T.-H., Lee, M.-H., Kang, K.-W., Kim, J.-H., Shin, K.-M., Lee, S., Jung, S.-Y., Kim, A.-R., Shin, M.-S., Jung, H.-J., Park, H.-J., Kim, S.-P., Baek, Y.-H., Hong, K.-E., & Choi, S.-M. (2023). Acupuncture for chronic fatigue syndrome and idiopathic chronic fatigue: A multicenter, nonblinded, randomized controlled trial. *Trials*, *16*(1). https://doi.org/10.1186/s13063-015-0857-0

Lan, Y., Wu, X., Tan, H.-J., Wu, N., Xing, J.-J., Wu, F.-S., Zhang, L.-X., & Liang, F.-R. (2015). Auricular acupuncture with seed or pellet attachments for primary insomnia: A systematic review and meta-analysis. *BMC Complementary and Alternative Medicine*, *15*(1). https://doi.org/10.1186/s12906-015-0606-7

Leung, M. C. P., Yip, K. K., Lam, C. T., Lam, K. S., Lau, W., Yu, W. L., Leung, A. K. M., & So, K. (2013). Acupuncture improves cognitive function: A systematic review. *Neural Regeneration*

Research, *8*(18), 1673–1684. https://doi.org/10.3969/j.issn.1673-5374.2013.18.005

Lin, J.-G., Chan, Y.-Y., & Chen, Y.-H. (2012). Acupuncture for the treatment of opiate addiction. *Evidence-Based Complementary and Alternative Medicine*, 2012, 1–10. https://doi.org/10.1155/2012/739045

Liu, F., You, J., Li, Q., Fang, T., Chen, M., Tang, N., & Yan, X. (2019). Acupuncture for chronic pain-related insomnia: A systematic review and meta-analysis. *Evidence-Based Complementary and Alternative Medicine*, 2019, 1–10. https://doi.org/10.1155/2019/5381028

Lu, C., Yang, X.-J., & Hu, J. (2014). [Randomized controlled clinical trials of acupuncture and moxibustion treatment of chronic fatigue syndrome patients]. *Zhen Ci Yan Jiu = Acupuncture Research*, *39*(4), 313–317. https://pubmed.ncbi.nlm.nih.gov/25219128/

Lu, D. P., & Lu, G. P. (2013). An historical review and perspective on the impact of acupuncture on U.S. medicine and society. *Medical Acupuncture*, *25*(5), 311–316. https://doi.org/10.1089/acu.2012.0921

Manber, R., Schnyer, R. N., Lyell, D., Chambers, A. S., Caughey, A. B., Druzin, M., Carlyle, E., Celio, C., Gress, J. L., Huang, M. I., Kalista, T., Martin-Okada, R., & Allen, J. J. B. (2023). Acupuncture for depression during pregnancy. *Obstetrics & Gynecology*, *115*(3), 511–520. https://doi.org/10.1097/aog.0b013e3181cc0816

Manheimer, E., Cheng, K., Linde, K., Lao, L., & Wieland, S. (2010). *Acupuncture for osteoarthritis*. Cochrane.org. https://www.cochrane.org/CD001977/MUSKEL_acupuncture-for-osteoarthritis

Manohar, R. (2010). *Ancient acupuncture techniques discovered in Andean tattoos*. Medindia. https://www.medindia.net/news/ancient-acupuncture-techniques-discovered-in-andean-tattoos-75007-1.htm

Montazeri, K., Farahnakian, M., & Saghaei, M. (2002). The effect of acupuncture on the acute withdrawal symptoms from rapid opiate detoxification. *Acta Anaesthesiologica Sinica, 40*(4), 173–177. https://pubmed.ncbi.nlm.nih.gov/12596615/

Morehead, A., & Salmon, G. (2020). Efficacy of acupuncture/acupressure in the prevention and treatment of nausea and vomiting across multiple patient populations. *Nursing Clinics of North America, 55*(4), 571–580. https://doi.org/10.1016/j.cnur.2020.07.001

National Alliance on Mental Illness. (2017). *Anxiety disorders.* Nami.org. https://www.nami.org/About-Mental-Illness/Mental-Health-Conditions/Anxiety-Disorders

National Center for Chronic Disease Prevention and Health Promotion. (2009). *The power of prevention; chronic disease . . . the public health challenge of the 21st century.* Stacks.cdc.gov. https://stacks.cdc.gov/view/cdc/5509

National Center for Complementary and Integrative Health. (2023). *About NCCIH.* NCCIH. https://www.nccih.nih.gov/about

National Certification Commission for Acupuncture and Oriental Medicine. (2020). *State licensure requirements interactive map.* Nccaom.org. https://www.nccaom.org/state-licensure/

NIH Consensus Conference. (1998). NIH consensus conference. Acupuncture. *JAMA, 280*(17), 1518–1524. https://pubmed.ncbi.nlm.nih.gov/9809733/

Pan, J., Lin, B., Chen, M., Zhang, W., & Lou, B. (2017). [Effects of tooth extraction under acupuncture anesthesia]. *Zhongguo Zhen Jiu = Chinese Acupuncture & Moxibustion, 37*(6), 643–646. https://doi.org/10.13703/j.0255-2930.2017.06.019

Pires, M. C., Barros, G. A. M. de, Fonseca, L. G. F., Thom, M. M., Junior, P. do N., & Módolo, N. S. P. (2022). Effects of preoperative acupuncture on prevention of nausea and vomiting and plasma serotonin values in the hysterectomy postoperative period: A randomized clinical trial. *Journal of Acupuncture and Meridian Studies*, *15*(5), 300–306. https://doi.org/10.51507/j.jams.2022.15.5.300

Qin, Z., Liu, X., Wu, J., Zhai, Y., & Liu, Z. (2015). Effectiveness of acupuncture for treating sciatica: A systematic review and meta-analysis. *Evidence-Based Complementary and Alternative Medicine*, 2015, 1–13. https://doi.org/10.1155/2015/425108

Shetty, G. B., Shetty, B., & Mooventhan, A. (2018). Efficacy of acupuncture in the management of primary dysmenorrhea: A randomized controlled trial. *Journal of Acupuncture and Meridian Studies*, *11*(4), 153–158. https://doi.org/10.1016/j.jams.2018.04.001

Shi, L., Feng, L., Yang, Y., Li, X., Zhang, M., Zhang, Y., & Ni, Q. (2018). Prevention of type 2 diabetes mellitus with acupuncture. *Medicine*, *97*(48), e13355. https://doi.org/10.1097/md.0000000000013355

Smith, C. A., Armour, M., Lee, M. S., Wang, L.-Q., & Hay, P. J. (2018). Acupuncture for depression. *Cochrane Database of Systematic Reviews*, *3*(3). https://doi.org/10.1002/14651858.cd004046.pub4

Sudhakaran, P. (2020). Acupuncture for hypertension using traditional chinese medicine concepts. *Medical Acupuncture*, *33*(1). https://doi.org/10.1089/acu.2020.1422

Urits, I., Patel, M., Putz, M. E., Monteferrante, N. R., Nguyen, D., An, D., Cornett, E. M., Hasoon, J., Kaye, A. D., & Viswanath, O. (2020). Acupuncture and its role in the treatment of migraine headaches. *Neurology and Therapy*, *9*(2), 375–394. https://doi.org/10.1007/s40120-020-00216-1

Vickers, A. J., Cronin, A. M., Maschino, A. C., Lewith, G., MacPherson, H., Foster, N. E., Sherman, K. J., Witt, C. M., Linde, K., & Acupuncture Trialists' Collaboration. (2012).

Acupuncture for chronic pain. *Archives of Internal Medicine, 172*(19), 1444. https://doi.org/10.1001/archinternmed.2012.3654

Wang, L., Xu, J., Zhan, Y., & Pei, J. (2023). Acupuncture for obstructive sleep apnea (OSA) in adults: A systematic review and meta-analysis. *BioMed Research International*, 2020, 1–10. https://doi.org/10.1155/2020/6972327

Xu, S., Yu, L., Luo, X., Wang, M., Chen, G., Zhang, Q., Liu, W., Zhou, Z., Song, J., Jing, H., Huang, G., Liang, F., Wang, H., & Wang, W. (2020). Manual acupuncture versus sham acupuncture and usual care for prophylaxis of episodic migraine without aura: Multicentre, randomised clinical trial. *BMJ*, m697. https://doi.org/10.1136/bmj.m697

Yang, X., Yang, N., Huang, F., Ren, S., & Li, Z. (2021). Effectiveness of acupuncture on anxiety disorder: A systematic review and meta-analysis of randomised controlled trials. *Annals of General Psychiatry, 20*(1). https://doi.org/10.1186/s12991-021-00327-5

Yao, H., Wei, D., Cai, D., Yu, S., Zhang, C., Wei, J., Xiao, X., & Zhou, Q. (2016). [Effects of acupuncture on ANP and CNP in adrenal gland and CORT in plasma in rats with chronic emotional stress anxiety]. *Zhongguo Zhen Jiu = Chinese Acupuncture & Moxibustion, 36*(2), 169–174. https://pubmed.ncbi.nlm.nih.gov/27348920/

Yeh, M.-L., Ko, S.-H., Wang, M.-H., Chi, C.-C., & Chung, Y.-C. (2017). Acupuncture-Related techniques for psoriasis: A systematic review with pairwise and network meta-analyses of randomized controlled trials. *The Journal of Alternative and Complementary Medicine, 23*(12), 930–940. https://doi.org/10.1089/acm.2016.0158

Yin, X., Li, W., Wu, H., Dong, B., Ma, J., Li, S., Lao, L., & Xu, S. (2020). Efficacy of electroacupuncture on treating depression-related insomnia: A randomized controlled trial. *Nature and Science of Sleep*, Volume 12, 497–508. https://doi.org/10.2147/nss.s253320

Zhang, N. M., Vesty, G., & Zheng, Z. (2023). Healthcare professionals' attitudes to integration of acupuncture in western medicine: A mixed-method systematic review. *Pain Management Nursing, 22*(6). https://doi.org/10.1016/j.pmn.2021.03.010

Zhang, X.-W., Hou, W.-B., Pu, F.-L., Wang, X.-F., Wang, Y.-R., Yang, M., Cheng, K., Wang, Y., Robinson, N., & Liu, J.-P. (2022). Acupuncture for cancer-related conditions: An overview of systematic reviews. Phytomedicine: *International Journal of Phytotherapy and Phytopharmacology*, 106, 154430. https://doi.org/10.1016/j.phymed.2022.154430

Made in the USA
Las Vegas, NV
09 July 2025

24662071R00066